Come Dance With Me

Come Dance With Me

Exploring the Body–Mind Connection

Judith Nicholson

LL.B (Hons)
Certified Practitioner
Rosen Method
of Bodywork

First Published in 2006 by
Ian Nicholson
26 Balcombe Street
Mornington
Victoria 3931
Australia
E-mail: thenix@ozemail.com.au
Website: www.rosenmethod.com.au

National Library of Australia Cataloguing-in-Publication data

Nicholson, Judith A.
Come dance with me exploring the body-mind connection.

Bibliography.
ISBN 1 920892 56 7.

1. Nicholson, Judith A. 2. Healers - Australia - Biography.
3. Mind and body. 4. Touch - Therapeutic use. I. Title.

615.851092

Cover and text design: David Constable
Typeset in: 11/14 Bembo
Produced by Publishing Solutions

Front Cover Painting

In 1991 I was fortunate to be one of Judith's clients as she was on the final stretch of her course in Rosen Method therapy in Stockholm. During seven sessions of her expert and compassionate treatment, we worked together to release emotions and feelings that had been packed down in my clenched muscles.

After each session I felt a compulsion to paint. My first effort was an enclosed bud like figure. The paintings continued until the dancing girl expressing freedom appeared. I felt that so many of my inhibitions had reached the surface and been overcome that I didn't need to stand back and observe – I could be active and creative.

Julie Vidal

Preface

I first met Judith in 1988 at Axelson's Gymnastica Institute in Sweden, the largest, oldest and most successful institute teaching my method of bodywork. She had come seeking a change in her life from law and diplomacy, relief from nagging back pain, and to further her interest in the body-mind connection. I trained Judith when I visited Sweden and subsequently met her when she visited California. Judith completed her training and qualified as a Rosen practitioner in Sweden, just before it was time for her to return to Australia.

Judith was an enthusiastic student with very sensitive hands and a perceptive understanding of the basis of what I was teaching. I had the feeling that she would want to import my method to Australia, and this she did. She established the teaching of Rosen Method in Australia, inviting teachers from Sweden and the United States. There are now six qualified Rosen Method practitioners and a dozen interns in training in Australia. I am proud of the great contribution she made to the spread of Rosen Method internationally and of the excellent partnership she achieved with one of my senior students, Gloria Hessellund, who became Senior Teacher for Australia.

Judith's account of her training and her explanation of Rosen Method are not the only subjects of her unique book. It is the intimate story of her life and of her attempt to understand and explore the unconscious mind and the body-mind connection. As a legal academic, Judith greatly valued the rational and persuasive power of evidence. She was also an admirer of Jung. In this book she undertakes an exploration of her own unconscious, revealing its influence on her life and the possibility of change that it opened. Through her clear and evocative writing Judith captures the challenge of this exploration.

Judith then tells the story of her three bouts with cancer and how she courageously dealt with them, drawing on her experience of the body-mind connection. Those facing cancer or other life threatening diseases will find comfort and assistance from her frank account of her feelings, of how she managed during those traumatic periods in her life, and of the way in which she contemplated facing death.

I admire Judith's many talents and she is greatly missed. I am privileged to introduce you to her story and am so glad that she has recorded such rare and intimate insights as a gift to all readers of this book.

Marion Rosen
Founder of Rosen Method Bodywork,
Berkeley, California.

Hindu India developed a magnificent image
to describe God's relationship with creation.
God "dances" Creation,
He is the Dancer, Creation is his Dance.
The dance is different from the dancer,
yet it has no existence apart from him.
You cannot take it home in a box,
if it pleases you.
The moment the dancer stops,
the dance ceases to be.

Anthony de Mello, S.J.
The Song of the Bird

It came to me one day that I was to live my whole life
so that it, of itself,
would be the most exquisite work of art I could possibly create.

Judith Nicholson, Journal, April 1991

Contents

PART I

Setting Out

I would like to beg of you, dear friend, as well as I can,
to have patience with everything
that remains unsolved
in your heart.
Try to live the *questions themselves*,
like locked rooms and like books written in a foreign language.

Rainer Maria Rilke
Letters to a Young Poet

Of a Sparkle, a Lilt and the Joy of Life

A*s you pick up this book,* can you imagine that I am sitting on the edge of a table talking to a group of people of whom you are one? There I am with my curly white hair and deep brown eyes, dressed as usual in blues, pinks and occasionally greens. You glance around the room, yes, others seem to be listening to me as carefully as you are. There is something in what I am saying that seems to be attracting you all. Or maybe it is just the manner in which I am talking: for there is a sparkle in my eye and a lilt in my voice. It is clear that I love my subject with a quiet passion and I am hoping to pass on some of my enthusiasm.

When you know me better you will understand that I am passionate when I talk of how my exploration of my unconscious, with its treasure chest of previously unknown feelings and associated insights, changed my life. In the early twenty-first century many people see exploring the unconscious simply in terms of counselling: on the one hand for those people who had an unhappy childhood, or for those who have just lived through an adult disaster; or, on the other, in terms of mysterious and expensive psychoanalysis. These seem to involve pain and trauma. So I meet friends and colleagues who say to me, "Oh I know I should explore my unconscious, but I just don't dare."

Similarly, when I was searching for a publisher for this book, I was told that people are frightened of the unconscious, frightened of the world of feelings, don't want to know about it and won't buy books about it. To which I replied, in tones of mounting frustration, that to debunk that myth was the very reason I had written this book. I want to tell people that this world of feelings is greatly misunderstood, that it is not to be feared, is not the prerogative of experts and not only for people in trouble. It is a world of great beauty, of colour and texture that can bring not only repressed feelings to consciousness, but also inspiration, insights, intuitions — and illumination of a previously unknown richness — to *the living of any life*.

I think it is the fact that it can add a new dimension to any life that people find so hard to understand. When I give talks I usually start by asking the people in the group, "Do you know who you are, do you understand yourself, do you know how you will react in a particular situation?" Then I ask, "... and if you do know, do you think you can change yourself?" Most people are shaking their heads by this time. However, in my experience, people willing to explore this hidden part of themselves can discover what sort of person they are and, if they find that limiting or constricting, then they can change. Not over night, no; but over time, and with plenty of love and compassion for oneself, most things can be turned around.

Let me give you one example. All my life I have felt the need to be good, to do what the majority in any group wanted to do, to act within established norms. I never understood why this should be so, I only knew that for me to act in any other way was extraordinarily difficult. And I simply assumed that this was how I was and would always be. When I did my training in the Rosen Method Bodywork — a way of contacting repressed feelings — exploring the previously-largely-unknown major experiences of my childhood, I unravelled this mystery. I experienced myself as a frightened tantrumming toddler whose mother had been absent in hospital for some weeks and whose carer was slapping my chubby little leg and saying "Mummy won't came back if you are not a good girl". Ah, so I had to repress all impish, adventuring thoughts and be a good little girl or "mummy won't come back" — a powerful incentive.[1]

Later, I also saw my life as an only child in a different light; I was a much-loved child living in a warm happy harmonious family. However, in that family, I had no peer group and it appeared that I never really felt as if I "belonged". I always seemed to be the odd man out, always striving to meet the approval of others, and to be asked to join their tribe.[2] There is nothing intrinsically wrong with always being "good"; but always meeting the expectations of others limits the ways I may want to behave as an adult.

Many of the feelings that lie deep in the unconscious are not well known, or if known, not well understood. I am talking now of creativity, with its helpmates inspiration and insight, of joy and passion, of love untrammelled by vulnerability and fears of rejection, of trust and of inner strength and courage. The almost unspeakable richness of a feeling that says I am all right just as I am, and I will be all right no matter what happens. Any of these, once experienced and understood, can add immeasurably to individual lives.

Additionally, many of these feelings can also carry a spiritual or mystical significance. I chose to wander into this world and found what I call the Divine and my passion for Life. That was my choice, it can be yours or not as you choose. It is a world of wonder and magic. The wonder of a beautiful rose, the glory of a summer's sunset, the strength and beauty of a forest of old trees. These feelings are unsuspected jewels lying deep within the unconscious and freely available to anyone and everyone.[3]

Recently cancer came into my life, not just once but three times over a period of nine years. This has been a tough time, no doubt of that. Cancer brought with it, however, insights into more new and unexpected feelings, paradoxically the freedom available if I could accept the immutable, and surprisingly, the quiet joy of feeling responsible for my own life. Last but by no means least, cancer brought me to face the reality of death. Death was suddenly and unexpectedly no longer simply an intellectual concept, something that would come to me sometime at the

---

1 See *Bendigo: Dancing Cheek to Cheek*, p. 101

2 See *Odd Man Out*, p. 253

3 See Part IV, p. 125

end of my life. But death, here and now, this year, next year, sitting at the end of my bed. What did death mean for me and how did that meaning affect the way I lived my life?

I have made this book a *case study* of what happened to me. Personally I am put off by speakers and writers who are vehement and aggressive in the pursuit of their causes. So I have sought to say quietly, lucidly, objectively and in as balanced a manner as possible, "Look I made an in-depth exploration of my unconscious using Rosen Method Bodywork and meditation to facilitate that contact. I went on to explore the body-mind continuum through the changes in my life and my three brushes with cancer. This is what happened to my life." I know my passion shows more when I speak than when I write, but don't be deceived. There is passion in the writing also. How else would I have had the commitment to spend nearly ten years of my life — with many interruptions — writing this book?

Thus *Come Dance with Me* is the story of my travels in the world of my feelings: first as I faced giving up teaching law and started to meditate, then during my training as a practitioner of Rosen Method Bodywork in Sweden, then on my return to Australia as the first and only (at that time) certified Rosen practitioner in the country. Later this world of feelings was helpful as I sought to establish the Australian Rosen Practitioner training program and finally again during my three brushes with cancer between 1993 and 2002. Away from Rosen support on my return to Australia, I used my everyday life and health as relevant metaphors to interpret unconscious material and to look at the body-mind continuum on a broader canvas.

Travellers write stories about their experiences and chatty, intimate letters to their friends. In this book I have done both. There are stories of my Rosen training, my travels and my family, and there are reflections or letters to an imaginary friend, chatting about the more intimate parts of my voyage.[4]

The book is divided into eight parts that in turn are divided into tales, reflections and letters. I always had in mind that some readers would not

[4] See *Dearest Friend*, p. 30

read sequentially but prefer to dip into those areas of particular interest. The first third of the book (Parts I — III) explains how I came to Rosen Method Bodywork and its basic philosophy — the connection between muscle tension, possible unexplained pain and repressed feelings. It tells of my exploration of the feelings lying in the forgotten incidents of my childhood during my training from 1988 to 1991, leading to my understanding of how they were holding me back and of their importance in the formation of my adult personality. This is basically the world of the body-mind connection. Later, as my contact with my unconscious deepened and broadened, I found myself exploring the world of the body-mind-spirit connection (Part IV).

In 1991 my husband, Ian, and I returned to Australia and prepared for his retirement after thirty-six years as an officer of the Department of Foreign Affairs and Trade. For some years, my meditation had been suggesting the idea of a completely new life — that of small scale farming for Ian, and a Rosen Bodywork practice, combined with the running of a "retreat cottage", for me. Hence our decision to move to Tumut in south-eastern New South Wales. We lived eight years (1992-2000) near that small rural town in the foothills of the Snowy Mountains two hours drive from Canberra, and tackled the totally new life of a small-scale farmer and his body-therapist wife — again with much help from insights and inspiration from my unconscious. Here it became apparent that freedom involves the need to make responsible choices (Parts V and VI).

Fate then introduced cancer — a different form of bodywork — into my life: breast cancer in 1993, followed by acute myeloid leukaemia in the summer of 1996-1997, and then, secondary breast cancer in the first half of 2002. Part VII tells of my exploration of the world of breast cancer, the connection I saw between that cancer and my personality as I had understood it to have developed as a result of my childhood, and of my use of my own unconscious material to assist my recovery.

Although I was shocked and frightened to find myself with breast cancer again, there was still not a strong probability of my death. With acute myeloid leukaemia, on the other hand, the medical prognosis was that death was highly likely in the short term — one to three years. Much of Part VIII, therefore, deals with how I used unconscious material, much of it in the form of imagery and intuitions, in facing the reality of an early death. In February 2002, I was diagnosed with secondary breast cancer that can be managed but not eradicated. The final tale in Part VIII tells of my continuing and deeper exploration of the need to live the remainder of my life on such close terms with death, and the realisation that freedom involves the ability to accept the immutable.

Writing a book has been an unfulfilled dream of mine for as long as I can remember. Sitting at my computer writing this, I have suddenly realised that one of the greatest gifts from my unconscious has been finding the passion, the inspiration and the skills needed for writing. I sparkle quietly as I sit pensively at my computer: what shall I say this morning, how shall I say it? This way, that way? Shall I be understood? I just love to be able to write. Ah the joys lying hidden in the depths of my unconscious... *the joy of life...*

The Elephant's Child

Fate made me an only child: my mother was very ill on the birth of my younger brother; he died, no further children were possible.[5] And so like many an only child, I peopled my life with books. One of my favourite stories was that of the elephant's child with his "satiable curiosity" in Rudyard Kipling's *Just So Stories*. He was just so curious to find out more and more of the world in which he lived.

As I write an image from my childhood floats up. I see myself as a small child walking up Toorak Road in Melbourne hand in hand with Pop, a beloved grandfather, the sun shines, my chestnut-red hair glistens, I am laughing, capering with the sheer joy of it all. I am going for a walk with Pop, going exploring, absolutely anything may happen, life is such fun!

That small child was born into a middle class professional family: my father, a partner in a medium sized firm of solicitors, my mother a trained kindergarten teacher. My childhood was spent in and around the Melbourne of the 1930's Depression and World War II: a quiet city where food, clothing and housing were in short supply. In 1938 my parents rented half an unsuitable house for one year. Eleven years later, with the war and its consequential housing shortages, we were still there.

Both my parents believed in good education: I was sent to Melbourne

[5] See *Bendigo*, p. 101

Girls' Grammar and then studied law at the University of Melbourne, one of only eight women in a class of over a hundred men. The War over, I went to the ballet with my mother, the opera and cricket with my father, played inter-varsity basketball, as it then was (now netball), with the Melbourne University team, sang in a small group choir, and swam, surfed — played — on the Mornington Peninsula.

Studying law, I met Ian Nicholson, now my husband for over forty years. On graduating he joined the Department of External Affairs as it then was. I completed my legal training and was admitted to practise as a barrister and solicitor of the Supreme Court of Victoria and the High Court of Australia. Thus were set up the twin threads of the middle third of my life: my marriage, in effect, to the Department of Foreign Affairs and Trade, as it came to be called, and my own continuing interest in law.

Foreign Affairs life is a hard taskmaster. Outsiders see it as a world of excitement and glamour: all that travel, all those parties. True, travel and entertaining are a part of it. The travel, however, is unremitting, two years here, three there, bringing separation from family and friends, struggles on arrival with a foreign language and an unknown city, hassles with sick children, different curricula, and strange customs. The parties are more correctly called functions set up for a specific purpose which may have little to do with the enjoyment of the participants. I am not saying I didn't enjoy that life, for I did, very much at times; nor am I saying I didn't benefit from it, for clearly I did. I am saying, though, that ultimately I found it both disruptive and stressful and it was initially my idea that Ian should take early retirement.[6]

Pattering quietly on in the background was my other life, that of an academic lawyer teaching, whenever Ian's home postings would permit, in the Faculty of Law at the Australian National University in Canberra. In the early 1960s that too was a demanding life: four young children, no home help and minimal child-minding facilities. I prepared my lectures while the children slept and taught on Saturday mornings leaving Ian in charge. Only towards the end, working full time for the first time, with the children in boarding school (necessitated by the Foreign Affairs'

[6] See *Turning Points*, p. 167

moves) or at the University of Melbourne, did I gain some confidence in that role. Earlier I had always been uncertain, doubting the knowledge and ability affirmed in my certificates of qualification.

As I look back, both these threads of my life allowed opportunities for my natural curiosity. As an academic lawyer, I liked teaching: I enjoyed opening up possibilities of new ideas for students. Later, with my children grown up I had more time to explore some of those ideas and hoped to write a book on the development of the concept of property — a long held ambition. However, it then became apparent that I didn't have the depth of legal scholarship required. I had spent too much time travelling the world with Ian.[7] Foreign Affairs life also, with its travel, its requirement that staff and spouses overseas be well informed about the country in which they were living, and additionally be able to speak knowledgeably about Australia, gave full reign to curiosity.

Yet when in the mid 1980s I started to meditate, to be more introspective, to seek to understand myself a little, it came as a shock to realize that no matter how much I may have learnt of the world in which I lived, I knew little of myself other than as daughter of, wife of, mother of, teacher of, friend of — a series of labels which described me in terms of how I related to others and what I did. Where was the intrinsic Judith Nicholson in all this, what sort of person was she? It was clear that a time was coming when there would be space for me to do whatever I wanted to do with my own life. How could I know what that would be, or could be, if I did not know what sort of person I was, what I stood for, what I felt was the point of my life.

Spurred on by my meditation I began to look behind these outer labels. Two things only were really clear. The first was my almost neurotic need to be good. I knew I had to be good, had to behave in the accepted way at every level, in every situation, and was always struggling to meet the expectations and gain the approval of others. To act in any other way brought butterflies to my stomach, sleeplessness and feelings of near panic. Now one of my daughters is one of nature's born rebels. I watch in amazement: how did I come to have such a child? And also in admiration:

---

[7] See *Digging for Joy*, p. 127

would that I had the strength and the courage.

Additionally, I knew I was unbearably sensitive; able to be hurt by the slightest remark unwittingly made in passing, struggling, often unsuccessfully, not to take helpful advice offered by others as negative criticism. In my earliest school report, written when I was about six, my teachers had stated, "It is a pity Judith is so sensitive". Later reports praised my efforts to be less so. Whenever I tried to define my own heaven, I knew immediately it would be a place where I would not feel these daily hurtful pinpricks.

Beyond that the picture was murky. Over the years I had been captain of the basketball team, secretary of this, president of that. It appeared others thought I had leadership skills, could exercise power. When I became the wife of an Australian Ambassador, a Lecturer in Law, Sub-Dean of the Law Faculty, and President of the Foreign Affairs Women's Association, many of the people with whom I came in passing contact presumably assumed I was a strong, intelligent, powerful woman. Yet I knew that in those roles I was often uncertain, seeking support and advice from others. Super-sensitive people who feel they have to be good find any exercise of power a minefield of possible hurtful conflict. I know that from experience. My so-called power was much more apparent than real.

In 1988 I gave up my teaching and accompanied Ian on a posting to Stockholm. Looking back I see myself as a bundle of contradictions and uncertainties — appearing to be one sort of person, yet feeling another. On arrival I could have taken up craft, canvas work in particular in which I had dabbled over the years, in-door tennis and swimming (the social life attached to a diplomatic posting), travel or spent more time with my family. Instead, a series of coincidences brought me to meditation, the writing of C.G.Jung, the Rosen Method Bodywork and a gradual understanding of the hidden quirks of my own personality. For the meditation and the bodywork led me into another new world, hitherto completely unknown — that of my unconscious mind. This I started to explore with my usual curiosity and enthusiasm for things new and different.

When I started my travels in this new world, I now realise, I had fairly simplistic ideas about finding freedom from the more limiting repressed emotions resulting from my particular childhood.[8] However, as my journey progressed, it became apparent there was more to freedom than just being free and I found myself exploring the relationship between freedom, choice, responsibility and acceptance.

Now, fourteen years later, I have discovered I want to spend the remainder of my life offering others an opportunity to explore their unconscious world if they so desire, and, in so doing, find what it is they want to do with their lives.

Choices continued to appear; would I start a Rosen Method Bodywork practice on my return to Australia? Would I set up a Rosen intensive program based in Canberra?[9] Would I write a book about my contact with my unconscious via Rosen Method Bodywork, what it has offered me, what it can offer others? And, more recently, will I extend that Rosen program to northern New South Wales and possibly Victoria. Questions, choices, answers, on I go exploring the small piece of life that encircles me. How I still love that elephant's child with his "satiable curiosity"...

---

[8] See I *Choose Freedom*, p. 39

[9] See *Rosen Practitioner Training*, p. 53

And the Brakes Failed

One hot summer's day in 1984, driving my little old Mini down a steep hill towards a busy T junction, for the first time in my life, the brakes failed. So what did this supposedly level headed, sensible woman of fifty do in this crisis? Took both hands off the steering wheel and yelled "help, help" at the top of her voice! I then averted the crisis in the obvious way; a combination of the hand brake and gear changes took me safely round the corner and pulled up under a friendly tree. I was though, greatly shaken by my own initial reaction. How could I have been so stupid, so absolutely nitwitted? I could easily have had a serious accident. It was a humbling experience.

The first consequence was a recurrence of *candida*, at that time in my life, an almost chronic, gynaecological complaint. Since over the years western medicine had given at best temporary relief, this time I took my problem to a recommended naturopath. I can see him now, sitting behind his desk, "*Candida* is often a stress related problem for women," he said, "which I can relieve with meditation induced by acupuncture needles. Would you feel comfortable with that?" That was not a problem, my mother had been having acupuncture to relieve arthritic pain for years, and I had previously had finger-tip acupuncture to relieve my sciatica when living in Hong Kong. Since I also knew I had *candida* whenever I was pressured, I accepted his recommendation.

Then he made a suggestion with which I was not so comfortable. A small medicinal dose of cannabis would assist the effect of the acupuncture, he said. If I planned to take it, I should prepare myself, be in the house alone, be in a quiet and lovely room, for often people made contact in some way with the cosmos. This would bring great peace, great healing and, as a side effect, there would also be an alleviation of my *candida*. As I write this now, many years later, I find it hard to believe that I took that dose.

One thing I discovered immediately, as soon as I returned home, was that I was very frightened of "drugs", and their possible effect on me. It was some days before I was able to swallow that one tiny pill. Again, it was a beautiful day. Ian was working overseas, I was alone in our bedroom with the trees, a view of the hills and the streaming sun. It was just as the naturopath had predicted, a cosmic experience of great beauty, great intensity.

In my life as a woman, I have conceived and given birth four times. Previously I had seen that process in physical and emotional terms. That afternoon it was as if I conceived again, this time in metaphysical terms. I watched a sperm enter and approach an ovum within. They were labelled plus (+) and minus (-) as for an electrical charge. As they met, I saw the fusion, I felt the charge, I felt the Life. I had a flash of instantaneous intuitive knowledge that was to transform my life over a period of years. As I experienced it, all life is a unified form of pure energy (currently unmeasurable by science). This energy is *Life*, *The Life Force*, and both gives birth to and comprises all things animal, vegetable, mineral or metaphysical. It alone remains when all else dies, it is permanent, enduring, Eternal. How long was I on my bed, thirty minutes, an hour? Not longer. I "surfaced" deeply moved and went downstairs quietly. Music seemed appropriate; I selected a recording of the Messiah and sat quietly listening as if in a trance.

The following six months brought great surprises, contact with a magnolia tree of great beauty, one in our front garden. It seemed to be "talking" to me, offering in some inexplicable way the strength of its deep-rootedness, the beauty of its pearly white flowers, the serenity of its glossy green leaves. Shocked, I took my experiences back to the naturopath; they seemed a little more than either of us had expected. He suggested a visit to Amy, the then Director of the Siddha Yoga Centre in Canberra, a quietly serene, softly spoken Scotswoman, overflowing with love, wisdom and compassion; she became one of my companions on my journey.

Dearest Amy, what must she have thought of the flustered middle aged woman, who arrived late one afternoon in her sitting room, with a garbled story of acupuncture, one small dose of cannabis and conversations with a magnolia? Patiently, gently, quietly, she listened, disentangled my story and replied. "Yes, she and many others had had similar experiences, in my case was I not simply living what I had already experienced on my bed that afternoon? Hadn't I said that I had then seen that all life was one? So now I was living it: I was "talking" to a tree; that was all right, many people had similar experiences." She looked and sounded so normal, so matter of fact, some of my fears receded, my life fell back into place. She suggested some books to read, a structure, a routine and a visit to the Siddha Yoga Centre.

Later, after my first visit to the Yoga Centre, I was meditating as I had now been taught. My tree was there and I was in touch with its spirit. Suddenly I heard and felt the words, "I am not only outside, I am also within, you and the tree are One". Then there was a prickling sensation as if small electric currents were running all over my body. Once again there was a flustered woman back in Amy's sitting room. Once again that same quiet, sensible, loving voice was saying this happens to other people also. That movement is the awakening of what the Yogis call *Kundalini*, the Life Force. It lies dormant in everyone awaiting the due moment of its awakening. There is nothing to fear, quite the reverse, you are greatly blessed.

When I discussed some of these experiences with a close friend well read in the catholic tradition, he suggested the possibility that I was becoming a mystic. I can see that scene now as I write. I am in a book-lined study, the sun streams in; the word mystic is in the air. Although I don't say so at the time, I don't really know what it means. Later I check my dictionary — someone who has a relationship with God. What on earth did this have to do with me? I was a fifty-two year old married woman, mother of four and law lecturer. I had had little religious training, no great interest in things religious, rarely went to church, and was dissatisfied and frustrated when I did. The word mystic seemed highly improbable, absurd almost. Yet, if pushed, I could agree it was connected with the various experiences that were surfacing from my meditation, but no great spiritual longing had carried me to that naturopath nor the meditation centre. I had gone seeking advice for the relief of *candida*; a chronic and exhausting condition.

Living in Canberra over the next few years, although I was frightened, confused and uncertain, something about the meditation drew me in. I continued my life with all its family and professional commitments, in all outward appearances the busy successful career woman of the 1980s. At weekends, though, just for a couple of hours, I meditated as I had been taught. I went only once or twice to the meditation evenings at the Siddha Yoga Centre. I never felt comfortable there: the incense, the chanting and music unnerved me. Amy was understanding and generous with her time, offering to see me quietly on my own about once a month or whenever I felt the need. And so our monthly chats, late on a Friday afternoon, also became part of my routine.

As we talked, Amy introduced me more generally to the writings of the Yogis — the Eastern mystics — their views that life was not just so many fragmented pieces all randomly knocking me about. Rather, life was whole, all of a piece, inter-linked. The key to unlocking the mystery of my place in this whole was to be found within myself. In the yoga tradition I was to go within, explore myself through my meditation.

Over the ensuing years, I have meditated in many different ways. Initially I sat cross-legged on my bed, as close as I could comfortably be to the traditional yoga lotus position, chanting the mantra which had been suggested. Later I began to meditate on phrases which I had read which seemed to carry an intensity all their own. Living in Sweden I came to have what I called my meditation walks, as I roamed the nearby woods with our German Shepherd, Sabina. Still later I began to concentrate on scenes of great beauty, to immerse, lose myself in the beach at Flinders where I had grown up, or that at Merimbula where I had had many happy holidays.

I have known others who lose themselves in music, poetry, or a favourite picture. Maybe this is not meditating in the yoga tradition, I am not sure, I don't know enough about it. All I do know is that for me I just need to let my mind quieten, become still, stop chasing the million and one things of my daily life, and that over the years I have done that in different ways in differing circumstances.

So it was lying in bed one night many years later, floating with ideas about my spiritual life, a sentence came up: *In the beginning was the Word, and the Word was with God, and the Word was God* — the opening phrases of the Gospel according to St John. Suddenly parts of my life dropped into place, as a jigsaw does when you find a missing piece: in the terms of the yogis it seemed I could be described, at least in part, as a follower on the path of knowledge; hence the attraction for me of things of the mind, the power of the word — in the beginning was the word...

This fitted with many of the things I knew of myself: my passion for books and reading, my need to find meaning. Over the years I have discovered I can face most things, so long as I can understand and, perhaps, have the semblance of control that such understanding brings. Without that I am uneasy, confused and, at times, close to panic. This is the curious Judith who survived many otherwise seemingly tedious diplomatic functions; the traveller/explorer Judith, whether in the physical world, or the world of ideas, seeking to understand more and more.

This is akin to the psychological process of "naming": once something is named, it becomes known, or capable of being known and so less frightening. Scientists, physicists in particular, explore the unknown mass of the universe, unravelling the mystery piece by piece, naming, describing as they go. Thereby bringing, say, quantum physics from the unknown mass to the known fragment with known characteristics. Similarly as I struggled with feelings of fear early in my meditation, Amy used to ask me to see an image of my fear, give it a shape, a name. My fear would become a black cloud or an ape; suddenly it was known, more manageable and less frightening.

As with physics in the universe or my fears, so with the ultimate mystery, the unknown X factor at the core of all our lives. In an attempt to name, describe, explain, the otherwise inexplicable, some of us use the word God, others The Guru, The Self, The Life Force, words all of them, carrying meaning for those who use them. In the Scripture classes and daily religious assemblies of the Anglican school I attended, I was introduced to the characteristics this branch of the Church had decreed should be associated with the word God. Here my personal perception grew of a fear-inspiring, perfection-seeking deity, whose worship seemed to be wrapped in dogmas and creeds I didn't understand and to which I couldn't relate. So when meditation came my way, it seemed I needed my own word to name my own personal experiences. In the beginning was the word...

I adopted at first Eastern nomenclature and talked of The Guru. Then I found that, too, unsatisfying: that word, like the word God, did not touch me, grab me, as a word must to have meaning in one's life. Over the years, I have tried others: Life Force, the Essence of life, the Higher Self; all happily used by others; all appropriate for me in some situations, yet not exactly my word...

As the years rolled by and it became clear I was developing a relationship with a beautiful "presence", my own word floated up — the Divine. Like a physicist exploring the universe I too began to name the characteristics of the Divine as they appeared to me, as I experienced them: Divine — unconditional love, compassion, warmth, vibrant vitality, clarity, simplicity, balance and finally after many years, sensitivity. In the beginning was the word, my words.

When I was living in Sweden, by a series of strange coincidences I spent a few days as a guest in a Benedictine Retreat House and went one morning to Swedish Lutheran Mass in the original Abbey church of St Birgitta. The omens were not auspicious: I knew neither the service, nor the language in which it was being conducted. Yet it was one of the most powerful experiences of my meditative life. I was, so my intuition said during the service, to be "a grass-roots" mystic, "a market-place" mystic, no retreat into a contemplative nunnery for me. I was to live my life as I had always done, showing by example that a deeply spiritual life was not a thing apart, but just one's own life with an additional dimension — an X factor, call it what you will. Moreover, added the intuition (as I watched the blackclothed priest, back to the congregation, address his God in his language), there were to be no intercessors for me. I had, was building, my own relationship with my own God figure in my own language; that was not only my privilege but also my responsibility.

That word *relationship* was fundamental for me. At Sunday school and in my Anglican school religious instruction and confirmation preparation, the emphasis seemed to concern what I was supposed to believe and therefore to do. There were stories to learn, prayers to say, dogma to understand, or more usually, to accept. No-one suggested that feelings could be involved, that one could have a relationship with the Divine just as one had relationships with parents, spouses, children and friends. Or perhaps if it was suggested, I was just too young and did not understand.

Words name things, differentiate one thing from another and so aid knowledge. However, in so doing, differences arise as to the precise meaning of a particular word. And it is sometimes forgotten that no definition carries real meaning for the hearer unless he or she can relate to it in some way: add their own feelings, to their understanding of that word. If I say I am angry, others have some idea what I mean, for they too have been what they call angry. Similarly if I talk of mystics and mysticism those words will carry for the hearers a meaning of which they have some understanding and to which they can relate.

Among the experts, there are differences about the exact definition of mysticism. Some people describe it in terms of the metaphor of marriage:

one is as if married to God, presupposing, a continued existence of both man, or woman, and God; the view of duality. Others use the metaphor of merging, dissolving, melting, into God, into the Divine. Life, all Life is then God, the Divine, one is no longer separate, as if married to and telling of one's experiences...one just is God — or the Divine. The view of non-duality.

I have found these differences unhelpful. All I understand is I am coming to know my own version of the Divine. This involves my being one who experiences and writes. One in fact who tells of what she has experienced. Even if at the time of writing I feel as if I have no separate existence from, am part of Divine...I still have to write as if I do; there is no other way. Once I take a fragment from the whole, and, using a word, I name it, then we have duality — me and the word I have used, the experience I have described. In the beginning was the word...

Now writing many years later, I look back in stunned amazement. The brakes failed in my car, I was stressed, *candida* came my way, I sought help from a new and very different source, although confused, uncertain and frightened, I started to meditate. From that one small incident on a summer's afternoon, the whole fabric of my life changed.

The Witchdoctor

Into a Land of Dreams and Fantasies

Flinders, Victoria, was for me, a place of warmth, light and security; a retreat, somewhere I used to go when the going was tough; a place from which to return to the outside world restored, refreshed, and able to do battle again. Here as a teenager I had wandered the beaches for hours watching the sea and the sky, dreaming, fantasising; there I walked the golf course with my father, and we had delicious cream sponges for afternoon tea; there, high up on the cliffs in a sunny grassy hollow one warm autumn day, Ian asked me to marry him and we set the course of our adult lives; here I took my family for long summer holidays, as I in my turn had been taken; here we swam and lazed in the sun — the lazy, hazy days of summer.

As I approached my mother's house in Flinders, it was hidden from view; then around a corner, there it was, tucked into the tea-tree, protected from the howling winds of Bass Strait. The front door was never used, we all entered from the back, straight into the kitchen: in front of us was a stunning view, light, sea, sky, clouds and the western head of Western Port Bay. No matter how fraught I was coming up the drive, the cloud lifted as I walked in the kitchen door: Flinders, for me was a place of loving protection, a place of healing and restoration.

I was staying in the house alone in the late summer of 1988. Since my mother was too frail and forgetful to continue living there by herself, I was packing up the house preparatory to handing it over to a purchaser. The air was fragrant with memories: curled up snug in front of a roaring fire reading on a cold wet winter's afternoon; the happy warmth of parties — our engagement party, Christmas dinners, birthdays, and the many visitors my father used to invite.

Now it all needed to be sorted — kept, thrown out or given away. By day it was the cupboards, tins so old they had no use-by date, thirty-five years of collected bank statements and cheque butts, old paint tins, pesticides, decades of clothes: nothing ever thrown out in case it "came in handy". By night it was the papers and letters — many pearls here: my father writing to ask permission to marry my mother; my letters as an eight year old evacuated with my school during World War II asking for boot polish and shoe laces; my mother's anxious letters in reply "are you all right darling?" To which it appeared she never had a satisfactory answer.

We used to say there were two typical Flinders days: when the cold south-west wind came in off Bass Strait, whipping up little white horses on the sea and whistling in the tea-tree; and still sunny days when the sea lay clear and sparkling like a polished blue mirror. Fate was kind in those weeks I was alone in early 1988. Clear sunny days succeeded one another; most afternoons I went pottering, idling on the beach revisiting old haunts, storing memories.

By Australian standards the Flinders beach is only fair: too many rocks and reefs for good surfing, too many pebbles and too much kelp to be attractive. Yet the rocks could be used for diving and you never knew what treasures you might find in the many rock pools. I had been lazing there one Saturday afternoon, swimming, watching the sea and the clouds, wondering what was to become of my life when Flinders was no longer a part of it.

That evening sitting cross-legged on my mother's bed, meditating, suddenly, unexpectedly, I took my first deep dive into the unknown depths of my unconscious. There I was, I could both see myself and feel myself — the imagery was very real. I was a North American Indian witchdoctor, a one-time powerful and highly respected shamanic healer. As I watched the scenes, I could feel my own influence, the awe and reverence in which I was held. Then there was a change of scene; something went horribly wrong. No longer was I respected and revered by my tribe's people, instead they were revolting against me and my evermore manipulative and abusive ways. I watched stunned as they chained me to a rock and left me to be pecked to death by the birds. I slipped down on the bed, curled up in a foetal position, threw my hands up to protect my head, and lay shivering and sobbing as the birds swooped and pecked. What on earth was all this about?

It seems unlikely, but as I recall, I slept well that night and woke feeling more curious than frightened. What had happened? Since I was alone in the house, but in any event didn't feel as if I wanted to discuss my experience with anyone, I spent a quiet day, reflecting and browsing again through *Healing and Wholeness*, a powerfully compelling book Amy had lent me that I had been reading and re-reading for the past few months.[10] In it I had met for the first time the ideas of C.G. Jung, the eminent Swiss founder of analytical psychology. In particular, his view that the conscious mind was only a part of the total me, that there was another part, the unconscious mind — a repository of repressed memories and repressed feelings — waiting to be asked to join the team.[11]

Looking back, it seems almost incredible that a reasonably well educated, well read woman of over fifty should have had no real understanding of the unconscious mind and its possible place in her life; but so it was. I had known in a scrappy way of the views of Freud — of an unconscious limited largely to repressed sexual desires — had felt them irrelevant in my own life and dismissed the whole subject.

Now I was reading that something called "the unconscious" was an integral part of my personality and could have a role to play in my urge to find out more about myself and my place in life. It seemed it made itself heard in a manner of its own choosing. When I had told the naturopath of my foolish shouting in the car, he replied that the unconscious often

---

[10] John A. Sandford, *Healing and Wholeness*, Paulist Press, New York, 1977.

[11] Book-lover that I am, I tried initially to read Jung's own writings, and, like many other lay readers was defeated by the erudition. I can respect it, marvel at it, but I cannot grasp it in all its detail. Therefore, like many others I have largely gleaned my ideas of Jung from the most accessible and reliable secondary sources. See bibliography for further references.

made itself heard in times of crisis. At that time I paid no heed, for I knew nothing of the unconscious and had no sense that I, as opposed to my brakes, was in need of help. Now, if I paused on that sunny morning-after-the-night-before at Flinders, here again it appeared was my unconscious making itself heard in its own way during my meditation.

On my first reading of *Healing and Wholeness* I had been particularly attracted to two strands of Jung's writings. First, he accepted the reality of a powerful independent autonomous unconscious in each person, an unconscious as real as the chairs we sit on, making itself available in our dreams and fantasies. Having previously spent many years of my life being told I was too sensitive, was often imagining things, or fantasising, it was comforting to read the possibility that my alleged fantasies could perhaps be my unconscious sending me messages that I was not yet trained to understand.

Second, was his view that in the depths of the unconscious, at the very centre of the psyche, was a controlling or pivotal point, which he called the *self* and described as the centre of orientation and meaning. This point, he maintained, comes into play when we seek to unravel ourselves from our past and discover meaning and purpose in our lives. Here again, echoing what Amy had told me of the Yogis, was the possibility that my life had a pattern of sorts, was not just blind malignant fate. It seemed I had been waiting all my life to hear that.

So I could accept my witchdoctor imagery was not just a fantasy; but rather my unconscious trying to tell me something that it felt would be helpful. Before I could unravel its mysteries, though, I would have to make sense of the imagery. It appeared from my reading that the unconscious did not communicate in words. Its language is that of pictures and images, which are symbolic for whatever it is trying to say — almost as if it is acting out a charade for our benefit. It depicts *what is happening*, not why it happened. Why, with its emphasis on rational and causative thinking processes, is a tool of the conscious mind. Seeking reliable and accurate means of interpreting unconscious imagery, Jung spent a lifetime researching symbolism in dreams, myths and fantasies, although stressing always that it was his client's association with any given symbol that was of prime importance.

Thus it seemed my unconscious had selected the image of the witchdoctor, that of a person of apparent power yet with feelings of total powerlessness and terror as he is attacked by the birds, in order to show me something. And as I had experienced this image, I had felt intensely as if all this was happening to me; if pushed I would have to say I knew it was happening to me. It was as Jung says, powerfully real for me.

At first, totally untrained in the symbolism of the unconscious, I interpreted the imagery literally: it was about a witchdoctor — a medicine man — so perhaps, its message was a cautionary tale about the use and possible abuse of power by people who sought to help others. Even before I left Australia to go to Sweden, it seemed my life was about to change. I suspected I would probably no longer teach law, would look for another focus to my life. I knew that helping others in one of its many guises was a possibility. Perhaps, I thought, my unconscious was simply providing advance warning of the dangers inherent in any situation where one person has power over another. With hindsight this was a simplistic view of that imagery, but it was the best I could manage at that time.

Later working with Ingrid in Sweden during my Rosen Bodywork training,[12] I came to have a more symbolic understanding of the imagery in the witchdoctor and to appreciate also that imagery can be interpreted differently in differing circumstances. I was struggling at that time with fears around independence in love. Together we looked at the witchdoctor and saw another message: that in so far as I was dependent on others for love, to that extent I laid myself open to be pecked to an emotional death by those others.

Total unexpectedness, being quite out of control, is a quirk of unconscious exploration; look at my witchdoctor experience. I had been happily pottering on the beach, I sit meditating and from nowhere the witchdoctor arrives. Gradually I learnt that my only control was to choose my means of access; then I had to wait and see what happened. Living in Sweden, I developed a deep and continuing contact by means of the

12 See *What's Happening Judith?* p. 81

bodywork sessions that were part of my Rosen Bodywork training, and in my meditation walks. I could have achieved similar results had I chosen to have more traditional therapy: some form of dream analysis or undergo a full Jungian analysis. Later, on my return to Australia, I chose to use both my everyday life and the pain and disease in my body as metaphors for the state of my unconscious.[13]

I think it probable that each person has an idiosyncratic experience of the unconscious. For me it is softer, more subtle, more diffuse, less clear cut and black and white than the world of my conscious mind. It is a timeless world of feelings and values, an eternal world where feelings greet one another across decades or even centuries, a world of synthesis, of bringing together many apparently disparate pieces to form an unexpected whole.

My conscious mind, on the other hand, having used words to express meaning, seeks to be more or less rational, analysing, differentiating and fragmenting one thing from another, making a structure from pieces clearly logically connected. Since I came under the influence of my unconscious, working with its imagery and symbolism, playing with the new ideas that came into my life, I find I have started to see previously unrecognised links and patterns and to make them into patterns which feel satisfying for me.[14]

These fundamental differences between the conscious and unconscious minds have affected the format of this book. Although when these experiences took place has largely become irrelevant to me, I realised this would not be the case for many of my readers who might find it confusing that in following an emotional thread I moved back and forth over time. I seemed to have three options. I could write a seamless web of reminiscences following the flow of the feelings involved and omitting any references to time; I could group memories together rigorously in accordance with the importance time has in the conscious mind, thereby losing much of the emotional continuity I was seeking; or I could try to compromise in some way. Since my unconscious travels have unearthed that I am basically a harmony loving person, I have tried to compromise:

---

[13] See *The Mirror of Life*, p. 153 and *A Broader Canvas*, p. 159

[14] See *The Heart's Wisdom*. p. 195

enough indications of time for a bewildered reader, not so many that I lose my emotional flow.[15] Bear with me on my at times erratic journeys.

When I read all my journals and letters from the preceding ten years in preparation for the writing of this book, I was dismayed to find I appeared to have been continually entangled in the same emotional issues, apparently simply going round in circles. Talking of this to a close counsellor friend she suggested I read the material again. "I think you will find," she said, "that you have seen new and possibly deeper aspects of an issue each time it came up. The voyage is not so much circular as spiral. You go around and then down a step, deeper down into the depths of a new world, gaining as you go new insights into the emotional ramifications of every experience."[16]

Writing about a spiral journey along lines in a book on sequentially numbered pages presents its own problem — repetition. One night dining with Phillipa, a close friend of long standing, and discussing possible structures for this book, she looked across the table, "I have an image for you," she said, " a patchwork quilt, you build your picture from a mosaic of images." "Yes, of course," I replied, "and of all the possible styles of patchwork, the one I find the most beautiful, is that where patches from treasured fabrics are placed, seemingly at random, yet a pattern emerges as if by chance as the quilt is finished." What follows, then is a patchwork of pieces, a mosaic of experiences and images evoking feelings. Some people will read it from beginning to end; some may just browse. There is some repetition, not too much, I hope.

And so it came about that with both Jung and the Yogis as guides I started to explore the world of my unconscious. Over the years I have read widely, and selecting an idea here and another there, have woven my own map as I went. In the writing, it sounds as if this were a conscious process, as if I made my itinerary, bought my tickets and set off. In fact, much of what happened in those early days just seemed to come about. I went to the naturopath, he sent me to Amy. I started to meditate, she lent me books, they interested me. I had my totally unexpected encounter with my witchdoctor and personally experienced the power of my own

[15] See *Idling*. p. 182

[16] See for example, *Point Leo* and *The Branded Little Soul*, p. 86 and p. 97

unconscious. A few months later I went to Sweden and spent four years training as a Rosen Method Bodywork practitioner — a person who is skilled in facilitating contact with the unconscious.[17]

Only now, many years later with the benefit of hindsight, writing a book about my travels, can I see a pattern developing clearly. It is not that I chose the road, rather it seems the road chose me. It appears as if the unconscious itself may have been controlling my journey, an example of the workings of Jung's *self*, coming into my life once I began to seek meaning and purpose.

17 See Part II.

Meet My Dear Friend

Dear Friend,

Hello, Friend — greetings down the ages, for it is ages, years, decades in fact since we first met, isn't it? Initially as I recall, you came into my life as a comforting presence for a small only child, in bed alone in the dark — an only child's imaginary friend. In those days I used to talk to you of my small doings, my hopes, my dreams, my fantasies.

Later at those times in my adult life when I was confused and uncertain, I used to wander beaches and parks talking reflectively to myself — to you my friend — seeking comfort, clarity and steadiness. Gradually, quietly, you came back into my life, a continuously available trusty companion: someone with whom I could be so open, so vulnerable, telling you things I would not dare to tell others for fear of ridicule or rejection.

And so in Stockholm, moving into the new world of meditation and bodywork, you became someone I used to take on my daily walks in the forests; someone I could talk to of the new feelings and ideas to which I was being subjected; someone who would listen quietly and compassionately. Someone who came with me on all my travels, who gave me a steadying hand: a friend, a simple word, a lovely word, carrying a depth of meaning.

Thank you for all your help, Friend, *please stay with me on my journey.*

In Limbo

Dear Friend,

In limbo, that's where I am at the moment, and a very uncomfortable place it is too. No longer in Canberra, surrounded by a group of warm supportive friends with whom I loved to talk, ramble, eat, laugh, work and play. No longer Judith Nicholson doing my own work, enjoying it for the most part, feeling I was making some contribution, however small, to the continuance of a legal system in Australia. Now, no longer enjoying the continuity, familiarity, stable security, small things that families bring into one's life: an unexpected phone call, a warm hug, a bunch of flowers.

Instead, here I am, uprooted, flung to the other end of the world, camped in a large, rather unwieldy house on the outskirts of Stockholm, miles away from anyone. Here, I am suffering rather worse than usual from the muddle, confusion, inefficiency and frustration of arriving to live in a city where one knows practically no one, barely speaks the local language, and somehow has to create order from chaos, usually very much alone. In limbo, certainly not in heaven, rather hovering on the outskirts of one of my own hells.

I am troubled by the travelling life I live with Ian. Today I am struggling with the loneliness of it. It can be very lonely at times, particularly when you are ill and in pain, struggling with doctors, hospitals and customs you don't understand; but also when you first arrive and strive to bring order to chaos. Here in this pleasant house all the equipment is Swedish made with Swedish language instruction books. The washing machine, a design such as I have never seen before, is a so-far-unconquered challenge, and is a twenty-yard walk from the kitchen! The supermarket is its usual lucky dip: how can I tell what I want, everything is wrapped in paper or opaque plastic, and I can't read the labels. Do I sound petulant, precious, Friend? Possibly, but I am unhappy; and I don't want to tell Ian. He has his own concerns as he struggles with new work and people in yet another post.

My dismay at my solitude may surprise you, embedded as it is in the endless round of social gatherings that form an intrinsic part of diplomatic life. I have often felt alone at these gatherings, because I did not speak the language sufficiently fluently, scarcely knew anyone, or did not feel drawn to those I did know. Yet to arrive in Stockholm in May as I did, at the beginning of the northern summer, is to be denied even that much company. Many Swedes are about to go away to enjoy their brief moment in the sun, as are most diplomats; diplomatic life is coming to a standstill.

I have lived with this feeling of being alone on arrival in a new post seven times before; it is an old friend, I know it passes with time. What I feel now, though, is something deeper, more confusing, more frightening. Not only am I alone in my large house on the outskirts of Stockholm day after day, but I seem to be absolutely alone — in limbo — in my life.

I have taught in the Law Faculty on and off since 1956 and, for the most part, enjoyed the teaching and the contact with the students. As much as anything I loved the opportunity to introduce the possibility of new ideas. In the last couple of years, though, I found myself irritated at times, losing patience: some of the students seemed so young, so naive. Did I really have to go yet again through the difference between a mortgagee and a mortgagor? I told myself this was grossly unfair to them and, if this was how I was feeling, then maybe the time had come to consider retirement.

When I began to meditate, I found myself looking at the legal system with new eyes. I can't now remember why I began to study law in 1951. My father had not pushed me. I do know, however, that later helping others to resolve disputes, trying to find justice was a big part of it. Perhaps I was just idealistic in those days, for by the mid-1980s, when I became Sub-Dean of the Faculty advising students on their subject selection and career opportunities, my perception was that many had chosen a career in law to make money and to help their clients to win at all costs. What had happened to justice?

Despite my growing ambivalence about my future, I had asked Ian in his posting preference form to request the administration of the department[18] that he be posted where I could continue either to teach law or at least do legal research. He was posted to Stockholm! Since the officially stated departmental line was that careers of spouses were considered in the posting of officers, I asked him to query this. Answer, Judith could always go to London if she was so anxious to continue her legal career. A quick check on the resources in the law library at the University of Stockholm and air fares to London, convinced me that circumstances beyond my control had brought my involvement with the formal academic side of law to an end, certainly for three to four years, and given the other uncertainties I had, probably for ever. That seemed to be that.

My father had been a Melbourne solicitor working quietly with people in need; the many letters written on his sudden death make it clear how much he was appreciated. I married a fellow law student who at times worked on the international aspects of law in the Department. Two of my children studied law, although one now uses the skills acquired in other fields. Thus, law in some shape or form has been part of my life ever since I can remember. When I pause and look at this now, is it any wonder I feel at a loss, uprooted as it were, in limbo, uncertain of my place in life.

The original "Binowee", my parents' house at Flinders on the Mornington Peninsula, has been for over thirty years, the one place where I always seemed to belong in my otherwise peripatetic life, the one place in this world where I felt safe and secure.[19] Now it is just a sea of memories passed to the hands of another. My mother, a frail forgetful eighty-four year old, could not continue to live there alone. We talked of it quietly she and I, such a painful decision for both of us. She would have to return to live in Melbourne, some hundred kilometres away, where she would have the support of close family. The house

---

18 Initially, the Department of External Affairs, then Foreign Affairs, later Foreign Affairs and Trade, of which Ian had been a permanent officer since 1955.

19 See *The Witchdoctor*, p. 22

would have to be sold so she could afford the accommodation she required. I spent the last six weeks before I came to Sweden, emptying that house of all its treasures, scrubbing it spotless for the purchaser. It was as if I was talking to the house: saying to it, we love you so dearly, we want you to look your very best for whoever comes next.

I know I talked about this before I left, Friend. How it seemed I would give up the teaching of law, sell my mother's house, pack up our own and give it to tenants, follow Ian to Sweden. In the talking it did not seem so bad: I had done it all before, could do it again, knew that if I lived through the first three months of any posting I usually came to enjoy it — some posts more than others. Yet this time it seems worse, perhaps it is the absolute finality of it all. I know I have given up law teaching now, not just for two or three years, but forever. Not only will I not see my mother in her kitchen at Flinders for a few years, but never again. It is these never, ever aspects that I have not experienced before which are so unsettling.

There is one last thing, Friend, it seems small of itself, but feels large. Everywhere I go I hear myself described as the wife of the Australian Ambassador: invitations come addressed to the Ambassador and Mrs Nicholson, I am introduced, introduce myself, described always in that same way. This has happened on other postings although it has never really worried me before, but now...Now I feel as if I have no real identity of my own, as if no one really sees me. It is as if I don't exist. In limbo perhaps, in limbo...

Thank you for being there for me to talk to Friend.

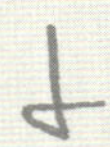

A Leap in the Dark

From Law to Bodywork[20]

Bodywork — the word has differing meanings for different people: panel-beating of cars to some, simple massage to others. In North America, where the Rosen Method Bodywork originates, the word is used generically to describe any method of handling the body that has as its express objective the facilitation of contact with previously repressed feelings held in the unconscious. There are a number of ways in which this may be done, of which the Rosen Method is one.

The word came into my life unexpectedly, unsought and, at the time, unknown; it gave me a new focus, a new direction, a new passion in life at a time when I was particularly unhappy and hesitant about my future. What am I talking of? What is bodywork? How is it able to effect such changes?

When I first arrived in Stockholm in May 1988, in addition to my emotional woes, I was in much physical pain: my neck, shoulders and upper back ached and burned. Previously, when living in Hong Kong, I had acupressure for the relief of sciatica — acupuncture but done with light subtle finger pressure instead of needles. So I decided to take my painful back to a recommended acupressurist.

---

[20] The following three tales are taken from two of my previously published articles: 'Changing Course: A Leap from 'Law to Bodywork', *Temenos: An Australian Jungian and Cultural Review*, Issue 2, Spring 1995, p. 44; Rosen Method Bodywork: A Newcomer to Australia', *The Natural Therapist*, Volume 13, No.1, 1998, p. 4.

The session developed very differently from my previous acupressure experiences. Inger, the practitioner, warned me that I might see images of my childhood, experience feelings, cry. What was I letting myself in for, I wondered? Should I leave, return home? But the pain drove me on, it was nasty, what did I have to lose?

Lying on the massage table, I was asked what was happening in my life that I was in pain. To my surprise I heard my voice reply that I supposed it was because I was unhappy. Then another question: what did I now want to do with my life, here in Sweden. As if from a distance, I heard myself unthinkingly reply: I had recently developed an interest in massage, had done and enjoyed a short hobby course in Canberra and had vaguely considered gaining professional qualifications in Swedish massage here in Stockholm.

That first session with Inger carried the essential essence of all bodywork: that there is a connection between physical and emotional states, that body and mind are closely interlinked: pain in one strongly suggesting the possibility of pain in the other, and most importantly, that feelings can be accessed through the body. Hear her question, "What is happening in your life that you are in pain?" Hear my answer — not the one from the conscious mind which would have referred to a strained back from moving house, hanging pictures, heaving books — but from the unconscious, straight from the body, unreflected upon, "I suppose it is because I am unhappy".

My formal session completed, Inger and I talked over coffee: she suggested my hands seemed small for Swedish massage, although they appeared very sensitive. She asked whether I had heard of bodywork, the Rosen Method in particular. My answer in a nutshell was "No", I had never heard of bodywork at all; but yes, I was interested. It was clear she had helped the pain in my back. It was also clear, as she continued to talk, that such work had connections with my developing interest in Jung and the unconscious. Rosen Method was taught in Stockholm in English, I was told, principally by teachers who came from the United States; language would not therefore be a problem for me, as it would be in other courses, such as Jin Shin Do Acupressure,[21] which were taught in Swedish.

A few weeks later with fifteen others, I did a four-day Introductory Workshop in Rosen Method Bodywork, and experienced my first formal Rosen Method Bodywork session. Stripped to my nickers, lying face down on a massage table under a blanket, I felt the practitioner's hands on my back: touching, probing, moving, gently but surely. I heard him tell the watching group of students that my right shoulder was higher than my left and that he could feel much tension in it. Suddenly he touched a spot as sore as a boil. "What's this about, Judith?" he asked quietly, neutrally. "Oh that's fear", I replied immediately, unthinkingly, in a matter of fact voice. Where had that answer come from? I had never made that connection before. What was happening that I was saying it now?

My session progressed with gentle, but nonetheless insistent touching of that tight, painful area. At first I thought to remain silent; why should I talk of my fears to a group of complete strangers? Yet the touch, though gentle, was firm, insistent, irresistible: it was as if I was driven to speak; slowly a lifetime of stories involving my fears tumbled out. Gradually my muscles relaxed, the tension eased, the pain receded and my arms stretched out further and further until, off the table, they were being supported by the watching group. Ake then remarked that I appeared to be stretching out to reach something, and asked if I knew what it was. At that time I gave what seemed an appropriate reply. With hindsight, it seems I may have been stretching out for more — for a new way of life.

Later when I understood much more of the Rosen Method, I could see that that first session contained its essential elements. Ake, through his handling and reflection to me of the muscle holding in my body, was able to bring about access to past feelings presently unacknowledged — my fears; and possible choices around feelings as yet unrecognized — the reaching out.

Four weeks later I enrolled at *Axelsons Gymnastica Institut* (the largest college of natural therapies in Stockholm) in the three to four year course required to become a certified practitioner of Rosen Method Bodywork. On a cold and windy day in early October 1988, with the threat of a

---

[21] Jin shin do is described by one of its exponents in the West as a synthesis of acupressure techniques, acupuncture theory, Taoist yogic methods and Western psychological theories. It places more emphasis on contact with feelings than the acupressure I had previously experienced in Hong Kong. See, Iona Marsaa Teerguarden, "*Acupressure Way of Health: Jin Shin Do*", Japanese Publications, Inc., 1978

northern winter looming, I entered a large windowless basement room. I was to spend many weeks in that room, and for me it came to symbolize the unconscious. I would leave the light of day, the warmth and security of my car, my known life, and go downstairs, down to what? Ah that was the rub. If fear of the unknown was one of my basic feelings, as it appeared, then the Rosen training was to give me plenty of practice in the handling of it. For I would never know from one day to another what the next training session would unearth.

On the very first day of our training, we were asked to recall ourselves as four year olds, and again as we had seen ourselves in the mirror that morning. I looked back sceptically, I had no previous experience of this sort of exercise, what would I see, how could it be of value? Suddenly, there I was at four, curly copper-red hair gleaming as I ran and skipped in the sun. I felt warm, secure and happy in my small world; I was vibrant, full of the joys of living, life was such fun, one great big adventure. And that morning, what had I seen that morning? The woman in the mirror was now not-so-young; she had steady brown eyes and curly grey hair. Her life had been free of the tragedies that some of her friends had faced. The warmth, the security, the happiness were still there, but there was a difference. It was as if I saw myself through a grey mist: I felt tired, burnt out, life was now a struggle, a burden; that spark, that zest for life and living which had been in the four year old, had faded as the years had passed.

It is difficult to say, even now with the benefit of hindsight, what drove my decision to commence and continue my bodywork training. It seems I was unsettled, uncertain about my future, open to possibilities, and when Rosen Method Bodywork came towards me it just felt right. Additionally, in some inexplicable way it seemed to be in harmony with my meditation. And so, I leapt, leapt away from the world of law and diplomacy and their known associations, leapt into the totally unknown realms of bodywork. A leap in the dark...

I Choose Freedom

M*any years later in Tumut as I start to write this book,* I walk the dogs down to the river with the words "I chose freedom" running insistently through my mind. I watch the phrase, play with it, dance with it; did I choose freedom I wonder, or was it perhaps that freedom chose me? I walk on, musing, and then sitting on an uprooted tree, watch the water gurgling and bubbling over the rocks, sparkling in the sun.

What are the feelings, the energy, that is driving this book into being? The word freedom comes. Yes, freedom, to be free, untrammelled, has always been one of the forces in my life. The word skips in the sun, shimmering over the water, a small simple word: easy to say, easy to spell, easy to think. I want to be free, will be free, a simple little word.

What do I mean, though, when I say that I want to be free? As a child I wanted to be free from the constraints of my parents: free to ride my bike anywhere, everywhere, to stay out late at night, not always to have to say where I was going. As young married parents Ian and I struggled to raise a family of four children with limited finances, needing always to be frugal and careful about expenses, endlessly budgeting. In those days I used to long for the freedom I felt more money would bring. Later in life with the constraints of parental responsibilities and budgeting more or less behind me, as a mere temporary lecturer (a situation brought about by my need to travel every few years with Ian) I felt the lack of acknowledged academic status as I struggled to feel free in my law teaching.

Later, bedevilled by cancer and its treatments, I found the prison of illness. Freedom it seems is always what we don't have! Indeed, one can apparently have everything and still feel trapped: the poor little rich girl.

Yet these are constraints of the external world; what of those we set ourselves, the limitations of the mind, both conscious and unconscious? As I look back down the years since I started meditating and Rosen Bodywork, that is where I have been — exploring, loosening the constraints of my mind. The bodywork took me on a journey of exploring the unconscious me, learning to understand myself, to unearth the patterns of behaviour I had taken on from others as a child; to see how these might be limiting my adult behaviour, and, wonder of wonders, realising that I could change myself, if I chose to be free…

There were tremendous opportunities for freedom for me here: to see what happened in my childhood that made me became a particular sort of person; to have the possibility of changing feelings that I no longer needed or liked. This is the possibility of being free from myself, free from bedevilling sensitivity, powerlessness, anger, addictive "busy-ness", the need to be good — to strive to meet the expectations of others or whatever else it may be. Freedom from myself, a veritable jewel.

As I gradually became free from myself, I was also free to be myself: free to find whatever it could be which would bring my creativity to the fore, with its pulsing vitality, its joy, its apparently limitless strength. I found it didn't have to be a dramatic or an artistic masterpiece. It just had to feel right for me and fire my enthusiasm.

The meditation set me off on another quest, that of my spiritual life. Here, too I found freedom, the freedom to follow my own intuition: to do whatever it was that felt good to me. It was, I found, not the Anglican church of my childhood, not even Christianity in all its aspects, nor Siddha Yoga; but an idea from here, a thought from there, a patchwork of pieces each one a part of the whole, and a whole that fits me and feels right for me. The gown of Judith, perhaps.

Meditation also brought insights, experiences of freedom in love, unconditional love; to try to love others that way, to try to love myself that way. That last one a veritable little ruby: to try to accept myself as I am, to say quietly to myself on hurting another, "It's all right, try not to be angry, remorseful, guilty. Take it quietly, you won't do it again. Let's see how best to sort it out now." To hold others be-loved, to be be-loved of myself: freedom in love, perhaps the greatest treasure of all.

As I sat by the shimmering river that late summer's morning, I saw where I had come: to a fundamental freedom, the freedom to be myself, and to do whatever that self needed to do with its life: freedom from myself, and freedom for myself. Did I choose freedom I wonder? Did freedom choose me? It matters not, for freedom it was that ultimately triumphed.

So, let us start out on my journey…

Shackles

Dear Friend,

What does my intuition want me to write to you about this morning, I wonder? A word comes instantly to mind: "shackles". Not a word that is frequently in my mind, or on my tongue! Although its mate, "freedom" has long been part of my life. Ever since I can remember two conflicting feelings have been pulling at me: a longing, a yearning to be free, absolutely free of all constraints; a terror of being rejected, of finding myself alone. A merry dance that pair has led me over the years.

What is the problem today? Why "shackles"? On the one hand I feel as if I apparently have everything I have ever said I wanted. That statement of itself gives pause for thought. Some imp murmured as I write "You are not supposed to have everything you want in this life, something dreadful will go wrong." "Get thee behind me Satan" must surely be the answer to that. And what is Satan, what are the shackles? Fear I suppose, fear of the unknown, fear of being so very alone, fear of this freedom itself that I have sought so long. Fear, one of the curses of my life.

And what is the answer to the fear, the shackles? I can see it in my mind; can I touch it with my awareness, can I feel it, make it mine? The answer is, it must be, trust. Such a simple little word, such a slippery, elusive customer. Blessed are they that trust, they will surely inherit the earth: warm, loving, joyous, carefree, spontaneous people. Would that we might all be ....

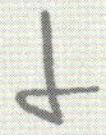

PART II

Listening to the Body

Even your body knows its heritage and
its rightful need and will not be deceived.
And your body is the harp of your soul,
And it is yours to bring forth sweet
music from it or confused sounds.

Khalil Gibran
The Prophet

Marion Rosen
A Wise Woman

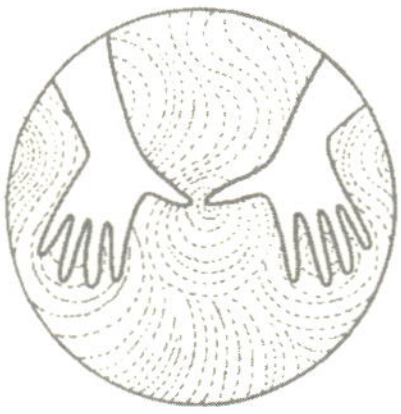

When I met Marion Rosen for the first time, I saw a tall, grey-haired woman, quiet, calm, seemingly a little detached, who stood before a class in Stockholm speaking softly, yet assuredly, of her work. The picture was not that of a powerful, dominating figure; yet there was a presence, something in her eyes, the tone of her voice, that drew me in. I wanted to hear more, move closer, be touched by her wisdom. Ah, that was the word I wanted — wisdom, I felt it in my bones; I was in the presence of a wise woman.

Marion is extraordinary. Born in 1914, she is still vital and vibrant, with the wonderful enthusiasm and curiosity of a child, and she continues to travel the world teaching, practising, promoting her Method. She is the living example of what she teaches: that life need not be painfully frustrating, can in fact be richly fulfilling, if we dispose of some of our past psychological baggage as we travel.

Born in Nuremberg, Germany, Marion first completed a two year apprenticeship in massage, breath work and relaxation in a clinic in Munich with Lucy Heyer, where these disciplines were practised in conjunction with Jungian analysis. Later she worked a further six months at the Tavistock Psychiatry Clinic in London, putting into practice the techniques she had studied in Germany. She then fled the Nazis before the outbreak of World War II, first to Stockholm, where she studied physical therapy (physiotherapy) and finally to the United States of America. There she retrained as a physical therapist at the Mayo Clinic, Minnesota, before beginning private practice in California.

For the next thirty five years, as she worked as a physiotherapist, Marion began to notice that, although she relieved muscular tension and consequential pain for her clients, many later returned; same tension, same pain. Slowly she realized that some, who had unburdened themselves during her work, talking of events in their lives connected with the tension, recovered more quickly, and in many cases did not return.

Gradually she developed an hypothesis, later to become the theoretical basis of her method of bodywork: that muscles used in expressing a feeling tighten unconsciously if that feeling is repressed or held back. Further, habitual tightening may render the feeling itself inaccessible. Thus the small boy firmly told that brave little boys do not cry, tightens the muscles in his neck he uses in crying (the scaleni muscles) every time tears threaten; if this becomes habitual, he may grow into an adult with tight muscles in his neck for whom tears are well nigh impossible.

One muscle attracted Marion's particular attention: the diaphragm, the largest muscle in the body and having both autonomic and non-autonomic functions relating to breathing. Her training at the clinic in Munich had introduced her to the importance of breath. Later as a physiotherapist she helped many asthmatic clients. Her second hypothesis developed around the relaxation of tension in the diaphragm and changes in breath. She came to regard the diaphragm as the interface between the conscious and unconscious minds: a change in the movement of breath through the diaphragm and the body, indicating a change in an emotional state.

The underlying philosophy of Rosen Method Bodywork is simple. Babies are born psychologically open and move spontaneously in accordance with the possibilities of their anatomical structure. Watch a toddler on the beach, see the open, springy, balanced spine, the steady, rhythmic breathing. As in the body, so too in the psyche: a tiny baby in a cot is trusting, open, self accepting. See that tiny baby ten, twenty years later, she[22] is watchful, careful, less spontaneous; the body, too, has taken its positions — stooped, braced, rigid, twisted.

Thus the theory of Rosen Method reflects Marion's experience as a physiotherapist: a muscle used in expressing a feeling will be tense if that feeling is held back; as that muscle relaxes and the feeling is contacted, there will be a movement of breath in both diaphragm and muscle. Stated this way it seems almost impossibly simple. Yet this simplicity is one of Rosen Method Bodywork's greatest strengths.

During my training in Stockholm, I listened to Marion many times. She talked of the choices that bodywork gives. A small child finds an incident painful and represses it together with the feelings involved. Sometimes the incident itself is traumatic; in many cases it is not. A harassed parent says sharply "don't make a noise, Granny is sick today," another, beset by troubles at the office, snaps "go away, can't you see I am busy." The small child, acutely sensitive to the tremors in her adult world, learns to be quiet, to go away, to do what is required to be accepted, thus unconsciously repressing her natural personality under a cloak of "shoulds" and "should nots". No blame is attributed to the adults: this was how they felt they had to be; no blame is attached to the child, this was how she felt. The purpose of bodywork is to reveal the incident with its holding, both physical and emotional. This done, the child now adult has the choice; either to suppress the memory and its associated feelings again, or to accept it and integrate those new-found feelings into her adult personality.

If muscle tension and breath are two of the fundamentals of Rosen Method, the wisdom of the body is the third: the knowledge and confidence Marion acquired over years of practice, to trust that each client's body will have its own deep sense of when and how to allow the release of its holding. Over the years she gained faith in that wisdom: to understand that although she may touch and focus on tight muscles or a movement of breath, the body itself is a unity, a whole, a being, and that wherever she touches, she is touching that being. The wisdom, in effect, to trust the innate healing capacity of a body and to allow it time and space. The wisdom of a wise woman.

---

22 Since babies are both boys and girls and Rosen practitioners, clients, teachers and students both men and women, rather than interrupt the flow of language with "he or she", I have opted to use either the masculine or the feminine indiscriminately. Although it is a fact that a higher proportion of the Rosen community are women, happily it is also a fact that there are men teachers, students, practitioners and clients.

Listening to the body, with an absence in the Rosen practitioner of judgment, diagnosis, or even a fixing attitude, listening to the body with attentive curiosity but no expectations, is fundamental to the notion of trusting the wisdom of the body. In Marion's view, to approach the body in a frame of mind which says "well, now, what have we here, what shall I do about it?" comes from the knowledge of the practitioner, and as such is likely to impede on-going contact with the wisdom in the body of her client.

Marion's aim is to be fully available, present for her client in a quietly curious, non-intrusive, non-judgmental manner. Her role is to facilitate through her skills, contact and conversation with the holding/wisdom in her client's body by means of reflection. If in this process the body is still, that too is accepted. This is bodywork, if the body is silent it has its reasons; she trusts its wisdom, she does not attempt to break down the holding. True to her beliefs, she honours even the silence of the body.

Reflection is the key here: to reflect to the client the holding in her body; to allow her to become aware of tensions of such long-standing, that they are no longer felt; to give her an opportunity to see her body as if in a mirror held by another; to talk to her body slowly, quietly in its own language, the language of pictures, images, signs, the language of the unconscious. It is this process of reflection which is one of Rosen Method's greatest strengths. It enables contact with unconscious holding in a body with minimal interference from the conscious minds of both practitioner and client. In particular it aims to free the session as far as possible from the distortions of unconscious projections, thus enabling contact with the wisdom of the body — pure bodywork if one can use that phrase.

When I watch Marion work she seems to match the tension/holding in a muscle with the pressure in her hands — no more, and probably no less. In effect her hands offer a non-verbal reflection of the tension, "look, you are tight here, remember?" A body often responds to this: a little sigh, a quiver, a tremor, an opening at the possibility of being heard, being understood. When she speaks it is of how she finds her client's body, keeping these observations open-ended, neutral, making it clear they are her impressions coming from a mirror she holds, not absolute judgments. "What's happening in the body?" she might ask, "how come you have to hold in this way?"

As her client begins to talk, she keeps track of the words used, not her interpretations or associations with the word, just the words themselves or their synonyms, and quietly reflects them back: oral reflection. At some point there may be a response in her client's body, a flutter in the muscle, a slight movement of breath, an insight: the tension, the holding in the unconscious has revealed itself. Teachers sometimes describe this process to students in terms of a midwife present at the birth of contact with a long repressed feeling.

Much of what she hears has never been able to be said before. It was too painful, too shaming, too humiliating; yet the relief with the telling is striking. We watch her client step down from the table, after what could seem from outside as a gruelling session; yet with clear eyes, shoulders back, head up, she says, "Oh I have never told anyone that before, it does feel good." She won't be able to speak, though, if she senses judgment, criticism, or even a fixing attitude (for that implies that there is something to fix). A quiet reflection is all that is required.

It is in this reflective, non-fixing, non-intrusive basis that Rosen Method differs from some other forms of bodywork. To see Marion give sessions is to be struck with the simplicity, the gentle, non-invasive nature of the work, at the same as one watches in wonder at its power and effectiveness.

As incidents/feelings/insights are revealed, it is clear that more than mere muscle tension is involved. A person may be deeply loving, but held back through fear of rejection; deeply creative, but frustrated through fear of assertion; delightfully playful, spontaneous, but restricted by the need to be good. During a Rosen session, she sees the way she, the child, decided she had to be; it was too unsafe, too painful any other way. That child was her own creation in that child-hood time and place. Now, though, the adult sees what has happened, sees the possibilities for change: the chance to be another person in another time and place, to remove a barrier.

Marion's gift to us all has been her willingness to accept the unique intrinsic value of each individual, to trust the body to allow that value to unfold thus permitting possibilities of change. Her work brings all of us a chance to move freely into the future unencumbered by out-dated baggage from the past.

Rosen Method Bodywork, the brain-child of Marion Rosen, the gift of a wise woman.

Rosen Practitioner Training

In October 1988 when I began the first stage of my Rosen training, Axelsons Gymnastica Institute on behalf of the Rosen Institute in Berkeley, California, required students of Rosen Method Bodywork to complete four ten day "intensives"[23] at approximately six monthly intervals, together with regular weekly day long sessions comprising anatomy lectures and hands on training.[24] The second stage, of a further eighteen months to two years, was an internship in which as practitioners-in-training we gave 375 approximately hour long Rosen sessions to clients, twenty-five under direct supervision, received twenty-five personal Rosen sessions ourselves from any qualified practitioner, and continued regular training sessions in small groups.[25]

The training was basically an apprenticeship, comprising demonstration sessions by the teachers on all students, the sharing of our experiences in this world of surfacing feelings, both in large groups and small, and hands-on practice. In every training session we watched sessions, gave sessions to one another, and at times, received sessions.

---

[23] Although I talk here of Rosen intensives in the context of Rosen practitioner training, participation in one or more intensives is open to anyone for personal growth.

[24] For a detailed discussion of Rosen Method Bodywork and training, see Elaine L. Mayland, *Rosen Method: An Approach to Wholeness and Well-being through the Body*, privately published, 8th Edition, 1996. In 1988 Elaine was Director of Rosen teaching for Axelson's in Scandinavia. She conducted intensives I attended, and was one of my two supervisors during my internship. She later founded and directed training centres in Canada, Switzerland, France and Holland.

[25] I describe the course I attended; *Axelsons* had versions for country students who could not attend weekly. Other versions have been developed to suit differing situations, as in Australia, see www.rosenmethod.com.au, subject to the standards of the Rosen Institute.

An intensive is what it says: an intense exposure to all aspects of Rosen Method. Slowly we developed the capacity to touch and be touched: to touch with soft, open, sensitive curious hands — to listen but not manipulate with our hands; to allow ourselves to be "touched" as we stood quietly by waiting, watching, listening, reflecting, being with our "clients" — but again not expecting, not manipulating in any way. In a supportive, confidential environment, we learnt to develop an atmosphere of trust and intimacy without which the practice of bodywork is impossible. Equally importantly, an intensive is designed to enable participants to move through their own emotional barriers or defences, to set in motion a process of self-awareness. As we did our intensives we went through some of our own psychological processes; clearly essential to avoid the risk of unconscious projections.

The only book theory studied was that of anatomy. We were required to have a knowledge of basic anatomy and physiology, a good grounding in the muscular-skeletal structure and larger surface muscles of the body, and thorough knowledge of the physical function of those muscles. A regular formal weekly two-hour class in anatomy was a compulsory segment of the first two years of my training. Although Marion refuses to draw a precise map of muscles and corresponding feelings, she does maintain a probability that a repressed feeling will often be found in the muscles normally used for its expression. Additional classes in Rosen or "experiential" anatomy, introducing students to the possible correlation between physical function and emotional content of the larger muscles, were conducted by teachers skilled both in physical anatomy and Rosen Method Bodywork.

The second stage of training, the internship, continued this same pattern only on a broader stage: we were required to give sessions, not just to one another but to members of the public, sometimes under direct supervision, always with the knowledge that a supervisor could be contacted. Our small group meetings contained elements of client review in addition to further broadening and deepening our own experience of the work.

Our own personal Rosen sessions were a vital segment of the training. Experience had shown the early practitioners that it was difficult to work with clients if they themselves were unconsciously holding in that area.[26] So as future practitioners we needed to unravel our own unconscious holding by means of Rosen Bodywork. It was recommended that we have approximately twelve sessions from one practitioner, not only to benefit from the continuity of working with the one person but also to experience a developing series of sessions; the remaining sessions could be from different practitioners. Thus these private sessions had a double benefit: as we worked through our own "stuff" we simultaneously experienced different working styles from different practitioners.

As I write (in 2000) there are thirteen training centres across the world, some varying the training pattern slightly to suit local conditions, but all subject to the standards set by the Rosen Institute which certifies every practitioner from every training centre. All are subject to the basic ethic: students need a good grounding in anatomy, muscles, muscle function and breath, for the rest this is work that has to be experienced and learned by experience, over and over again — experiential training. When I returned to Australia in 1991 with my certificate from the Rosen Institute in my luggage, I was the only Rosen Method practitioner in the country. As I set up my own practice in Tumut and Canberra with the nearest help in California, I realised just how thorough my training had been, and I blessed those inspired early Rosen practitioners who had devised it and taught me.

[26] This is common in most forms of therapy. Hence most well trained counsellors and therapists have a thorough knowledge of their own "stuff" and have regular peer supervision.

Being With…, Not Doing To…

At the beginning of my training, handicapped as I was by my almost total lack of Swedish, I told myself one of the things I must learn was to communicate with people in a new way. As Inger had said, the language of instruction in the intensives, the formal classes, was English, with translation for those few Swedes who needed it. However, in small groups, working in pairs, all anatomy classes, coffee and lunch breaks, most socialising was in Swedish. In my Foreign Affairs life, I had spent many hours drinking tea, smiling, pointing, miming, relating to people with whom I could not easily speak. Now I was doing it again, in another setting, sitting quietly in the basement at *Axelsons*, sharing coffee and companionship.

Anatomy classes were different. At first, I was recommended to an English language anatomy text used in the United States of America; however, our teachers were teaching from Swedish material. There were differences in content and emphasis that made it essential I follow their text. Soon most of my Government-funded Swedish lessons were taken up with anatomy translations. My tutor was not amused, she wanted the subjunctive, verbal moods and tenses, where she felt at home; not a struggle with the technical language of anatomy and physiology, where she certainly did not.

Once the extent of my plight became known, *Axelsons* appointed Ann-Margret as my translator, specifically for anatomy and the weekly small group training, but also casually in intensives, where she was often present as a class assistant and sometimes as a translator for the American teachers. Together we patiently negotiated the minefield of anatomy, comparing the English and Swedish texts, both of us learning as we went. She translated my exam papers which I was allowed to answer in English.

In class, giving and receiving sessions, it was as if Ann-Margret was my guardian shadow: she would appear as if by magic if I had language difficulties. From across the room she would catch my eye as I looked up and materialise right there beside me, "Are you all right Judith, do you need help?" In fact everyone, fellow students, teachers, assistants, *Axelsons Gymnastica Institut* (which I assumed paid Ann-Margret for her formal help) came to my aid with such ease, such friendship that I was deeply touched. It was both moving and humbling to be offered so much help with such grace and generosity.

Now as I look back I see in that generosity elements of the intangibles of Rosen Method Bodywork: to be met, welcomed and trusted just exactly as I was, a person, about whom no one knew anything and with whom some couldn't even communicate. This I now know is the essence of the work, what we were to absorb by osmosis during this experiential training — the simple meeting of one person, one human being by another free from conditioning and distortions. This meeting was brought about by touch, so that even those of us who could not readily communicate by speech came together. A meeting of the wisdom of one body with that of another.

To bring about such an open, judgment-free meeting, we were asked to "be with" our clients, to wait patiently while the body in its wisdom allowed a feeling to surface. "Being with", accepting "what is", involved a fundamental change in personal orientation, a total shift in how most of us had previously related to others, and more importantly to ourselves. This sat uneasily with almost every attitude most of us had as late twentieth century people. We had lived our lives asking consciously or unconsciously is this right, is this wrong, how can I fix it, please fix it for me — impliedly doing, working towards outcomes. Now we were being asked to put aside expectations as to outcomes, judgments as to right and wrong, to make no diagnosis as to why that might be and, in particular, to have no attitude that we were required to fix anything. It was an enormous change in attitude. We were, it appeared, to be curious facilitators of a meeting between our client and the holding in his body: midwives present at the birth of a repressed feeling.

For all of us this subtle shift in attitude came about slowly over a long period of time. Even now, many years later I can still slip here: an intuitive client said to me recently, "I sometimes have a whisp of a feeling that you want something for me." She was right, I saw it immediately: consciously or unconsciously I did; she is a gifted person so I want her to move past the blockage that appears to be holding her back. Yet wanting people to move to such an extent that I try to move them, is not my role as a Rosen practitioner. Accepting and reflecting, "being with", not "doing to"...

Physically, this "being with" involves listening to our client's body; learning to work with soft hands that formed an integral part of our skills training. In giving sessions, we were told, our hands should be soft, relaxed, sensitive, open and curious. In Marion's words we were touching, meeting the holding, bringing it once more into the conscious awareness of our "client", but not doing anything to it. It was as if touch was a new and beautiful bridge across which we walked to meet our clients in a different way.

"You have thousands of nerve endings in your hands," a visiting teacher said one morning, "use them to listen to your client's body." Listening to one's client's body, hearing and then reflecting the subtle nuances as the breath changes, a muscle flutters, or the body vibrates for a split second responding to a phrase that is powerful for it.

"Do you feel that response?" One of the assistants asked early in my training, as she helped me work on a fellow student? I nodded wordlessly; I had felt the response, but as yet could hardly credit it. Had I really felt that flutter under my fingers? I had made a general observation that the muscles on which I was working often tighten in situations in which one is holding back. Suddenly at the words "holding back", there had been a "fizz", a flutter, the slightest of vibrations in the body of my training partner, as if it were saying "yes, yes this is what this is all about", and simultaneously a trace of movement as breath came into a previously still area.

Slowly I learned to trust my ability to feel this response; to distinguish those situations where the body unexpectedly responded to a chance, seemingly irrelevant remark, and others where my partner would say something she already knew in her conscious mind and thought was important, and yet her body responded not one jot. Once experienced the power of this bodily response is undeniable. If it is present the remark is important; if it is absent the remark is unimportant in itself, although the fact that the mind thinks that it is important may be relevant.

Despite my language hassles, I felt immediately at home when it came to touching, listening with soft, sensitive hands. I had always been dimly aware that touching and texture were important to me, that I would stretch out to touch, to stroke, to feel in order to know. My hobbies in a very full life had been sewing, knitting, canvas work, feeling the threads, the fabric in my fingers: a tactile person, perhaps, but previously largely unrecognised as such.

Not only were we to have soft open hands, but also what one of my own students once beautifully described as "soft eyes". Eyes which were quietly aware of the whole body, able to pick up a flutter of movement in a leg while apparently working on a shoulder; not eyes which fiercely focussed, concentrated on one point to the exclusion of all others.

However, "being with" involved much more than listening with a soft physical touch and watching with soft eyes. We were also to be psychologically with our clients; different teachers as they spoke of this emphasised differing aspects of the work. Some talked of being a container for our clients, providing a safe certain place in which they could dare to meet long repressed feelings. Others spoke of being a companion on their journey standing quietly beside them, listening to what was said, a witness for them, affirming what had happened.

On the one hand we were to allow ourselves to relate to, be moved by their stories, yet, we were not to become entangled in them. Although I found, as I think we all did, the boundary between being moved by, but not enmeshed in, difficult at first, I loved the work. Buried under my legal training and the habits of a long life often spent with strangers in formal settings in foreign countries, I discovered another person, one who loved to be allowed to draw near to others, to talk of intimate things, to be trusted and to trust in turn. This came as a complete surprise. It was as if I met a part of myself I had never previously known.

The one further characteristic required in the work I knew I had — curiosity: I am innately curious, I just love to explore. Like many an only child, I peopled my life with books: lived the life of the Swallows and Amazons, sailed, camped, explored with John, Susan, Nancy and Peggy, found in their adventures and those of many others all the warmth, companionship and excitement of my missing brothers and sisters. Similarly as an academic lawyer, I loved to explore the world of ideas, teaching, opening up possibilities for students. Integrally involved in Marion's "being with", was a curiosity, an intention to explore the holding of a client, its boundaries, its depth and intensity: an intention present in both practitioner and client. It is as if we are knocking on the door of the holding: "Hello", we say, "there is holding here, can you tell me what happened that you have to hold in this way?"

There were about fifty-five of us in *Axelsons* basement, men and women, ranging in age from about thirty to sixty. We seemed to come from all walks of life: cooks, clerks, administrative assistants, nurses, teachers, massage therapists and, as I remember, only two therapists. In an infinite number of ways, I think most of us were curious, exploring, searching for something more to life: better relationships, more interesting work — not necessarily as Rosen practitioners[27] — less physical pain. Additionally perhaps, another common thread uniting all of us was the desire to touch and be touched in turn — both physically and psychologically. Perhaps it was as unconscious for the others as it had been for me.

---

[27] Some people attend Rosen intensives for personal growth. They then leave a program as they feel more certain of themselves and what they would like to attempt to do with their lives. Some of my fellow students left the program after one or two intensives.

Student life in the basement involved being clients as well as trainee-practitioners. In every training day, be it an intensive or a regular small group training, hearing the cry "pick a partner", we would work in pairs, each of us giving and receiving a session. Looking back I see real conflict for myself here. On the one hand my first Rosen session with Ake had established fear of the unknown as one of my basic feelings. Consequently, it seemed I was one of life's organisers, a maker of lists, crossing out, ticking off as I went, someone who was trying to feel in control of her life with less of the unknown to fear. Yet on the table I had no control over the content of a session. On the other hand, there was the relief in being met with soft yet undemanding hands, by someone who would listen to me and make no judgments, the relief of just being myself.

At first, I think, it was the relief in the absence both of judgment and expectations I found so compelling. No one was expecting me to be good, sensible or strong; no one was judging me as second rate or inadequate — so long as I did not make these judgments myself, of course. Later as I realised how much of my childhood I had spent feeling others were too preoccupied to have time for me, it was the fact of knowing someone was there to listen. And then, of course, that innate curiosity just drove me on, what sort of person was I...?

It was soon clear that the emotional sensitivity of which I had long known, was both a strength and a burden. It was so easy for me to make contact with my repressed feelings during an intensive, that by the end of ten days I was often both emotionally and physically exhausted — reduced to lying crying on my bed. When I developed shingles, it seemed I might be asked to give up the training. I was, it was said, too sensitive, could too easily take on the feelings of others to the detriment of my own health. Ironically, it seemed, the work could possibly be dangerous for someone as gifted for it as I appeared to be. In the end I took leave of absence for some months. Then on return, I focussed myself determinedly on reflection, detachment and compassion, the quality of being completely present as a person with another person, without becoming personally involved in anyway — "being with...'

And so for three years student life went on in *Axelsons* basement. We acquired our skills, learnt anatomy, gradually shifted from doing, fixing mode, to listening, "being with" and slowly discovered just what had happened that we had become as we were. It was probably the most challenging, yet exciting period of my life. At times I returned home to tell Ian I was quitting, it was all just too difficult, but I never did. There was something about it, something that came from nowhere that grabbed me and said, "this is you."

Walking in the Woods

Life as a Trainee-Client

Fear, fear of the unknown, the first feeling to surface from my body in that first Rosen session with Ake, is one of the deepest and most abiding feelings I found in my Rosen training. It is here with me today as I write: I have never written a book before, am not sure what is involved; do I have the skills, the creative ability, the clarity of thought, the language, the drive to bring it all together? I felt a sense of panic, I can't handle it and feel quite out of control. Here I meet another of my deeply held feelings — the diabolically demoralising feeling that, in whatever situation I might find myself, I just can't cope.

An image surfaced in an early Rosen session: it was March 1942, I was eight years old and three weeks previously had started a new school with four little friends from my former prep school. World War II was blazing away; Singapore had just fallen. The Royal Australian Air Force having unexpectedly requisitioned my new school with its many facilities in inner Melbourne, the school was to be evacuated to Marysville in the foothills, 120 kilometres away. Boarding school for a little eight-year-old only child, who as far as she could remember, had never before left her mother. In that Rosen session I saw an image of my mother in my bed the night before I left, she was comforting, soothing me, I would be all right, she said, I just had to trust her, she knew I would be all right.

Then I saw myself the following day going over a continuously winding mountain road, clutching my gas mask, separated by chance from my little friends and my possessions, vomiting out the car window. I felt the absolute terror and panic of a small child away from family and friends, quite out of control, and with absolutely no idea what will happen next. I realised as I saw that image almost fifty years later, why I had been driven to struggle with lists, boxes and inventories in all the twenty-two moves of our adult life, trying to stay in control; in Ian's view unnecessarily doing much of the professional packers' work. Ah, but I was the one carrying in my unconscious the hidden terrors of that evacuation to Marysville.

The Rosen teachers who interviewed me in Stockholm before I did my first intensive, said they did not doubt my suitability for the work, but were concerned that, since I had just arrived, I would not have a peer support network of family and friends. How would I find being so alone, they asked, with the possible de-stabling effect of surfacing feelings? In all innocence I replied that for over thirty-five years Ian and I had supported each other through all the vicissitudes of our travelling, family and professional lives; and so long as I had his support, I was sure I could manage. "Of course I'll help," he said when I asked, "if you are sure this is what you want to do." And, in fact, when at the end of the first week of my first intensive, I said it was all just too much and I would have to quit, my support person eased me back again. "You can't drop out now," he said, "you have only just begun."

And so it was that I set out on the other side of my Rosen training, that of being a trainee-client, having the work done to me over and over again, by my fellow students in practice sessions, by teachers in demonstration sessions, and finally by the Rosen practitioners who gave me my twenty five private personal sessions in my internship. The purpose of this was to give all of us repeated opportunities as practitioners for hands on practice, and as clients to make contact with our own feelings.

An additional advantage was that, as we sat sharing our feelings, we saw for ourselves the effects of the bodywork on one another. When I returned to Australia and was greeted by many sceptics, I could be quietly confident: I knew it worked, I had experienced it for myself, and seen it work for others.

Implicit in being a client, is an agreement to trust the innate healing capacity of the body, to listen to the wisdom of the body and, most importantly, to allow it to have control of when and what feelings "come up" in a session. As students we were advised not to "consciously release" feelings, not to act them out during a session. In Marion's view "acting out" inhibits contact with what is actually coming up. Thus the control of the content of a session is within the sphere of the body and through it the unconscious. The client's only conscious control is the option of terminating a session, a simple matter of sitting up and returning to the present.[28] As a receiver of Rosen sessions I have chosen to do this only once, and then I did not so much stop, as interrupt my session. In essence then, a client also is curious but without expectations as to the outcome of any session.

Even in that first intensive I discovered that my feelings were not as repressed as those of many of the Swedish students. My feelings started surfacing almost immediately and I began to feel badly in need of guidance and support which did not appear to be forthcoming. Although critical to myself at the lack of support offered by those conducting the intensive, I was too hesitant to raise the matter given my language difficulties and the unfamiliar situation.

Only much later did I realize that Rosen Method Bodywork was about facilitating contact with feelings and not professional help with their integration; this was the role of a counsellor or therapist. Later it appeared that, when during my first intensive, Lisen (a Swedish teacher) had given me the name of a counsellor to help me with the integration of the Rosen work and my meditation, she had expected I would see this counsellor on a regular basis. In fact I sought her help only once during that first intensive and never thought to see her again. In the early 1980s Australians of my

[28] All new clients are screened: people with drug, and alcohol related problems are unsuited to this form of therapy; people under psychiatric care need permission from their doctors, or their counsellors; people with physical injuries, torn ligaments and so on, should seek the appropriate medical care elsewhere; people with unexplained lumps or physical pain, should have them checked out with the usual medical tests.

generation were both ignorant and wary of counsellors. Now I realised I was in the very situation about which I had been warned: despite Ian's help, I was feeling very much alone and confused by all these surfacing feelings.

Searching for support in books, I read that if I was making contact with my unconscious, I should work with my hands in some way to help me express and integrate my newly discovered feelings. I should draw, paint, do clay modelling, use colours, shapes, imagery, symbols, the language of the unconscious. Given the foreign nature of the unconscious world in which I was travelling, I had no wish to enter other unknown worlds by drawing or painting. Despite warnings that the world of words could take me back to the conscious mind, I took to talking to myself, journalling and writing. It felt good to stay in a known world, the world of words where I felt very much at home. With four children living in Australia and international phone calls almost prohibitively expensive until quite recently, letter writing was something I had done naturally for years over many hours each week. And so I began my letters to my imaginary dear friend.

The many forests near our house were extraordinarily beautiful: almost deserted during the week, quiet and still with huge old conifers, mossy rocks and in some, sparkling blue lakes. Sabina, a most beautiful, strong, sensitive, German Shepherd — my greatest joy and the fulfilment of a long-held dream — used to take me for a walk in these forests everyday for at least an hour or two: if by mid-afternoon I had not suggested a walk, Sabina would be at the front door whining.

Once I started my Rosen training, I used these walks not only for musing and reflecting on the incidents and feelings which were coming up from my childhood, but also for floating, drifting, in the beauty of the countryside. And so these walks, part reflection, part meditation, became an integral part of every day, an inseparable part of my Rosen experience and my meditative life. As the months passed I found different walks to suit my every mood: one through flat even countryside when I was feeling too disturbed to pick my way, others with rocky more awkward paths when I was feeling more adventurous.

So it was that I was walking one day reflecting about fear. If I were giving a lecture in Property Law, I said to myself, I would be telling the students there were three ways of disposing of unwanted property: selling it, giving it away, or abandoning it. Yet, if I turn to my fear of which I now wished to dispose, I can't sell it, no fool would buy it; I can't give it away (absolutely no one would want it as a gift), that leaves abandonment. I was about to fling it away happily by the side of the road when a thought came: someone might find it and pick it up; it could be someone who was dear to me, I wouldn't want that. I paused. On reflection I found there was no one friend or foe, I wanted to have this fear. It seemed to be mine; somehow I had to learn to handle it and all the other feelings that came up in my training. Having chosen to contact them, their integration in my life was my responsibility and mine alone.[29]

It seems appropriate that since I was learning bodywork, it was the wisdom of my body, as it came from my meditation and my intuition, which helped me set up a basic support framework. I remembered that in the early days of my meditation, Amy had counselled against thinking too much about the thoughts and feelings which came up, "Just let them alone, Judith, let them come and go," she used to say, "watch them as an observer, a witness, but try to stay as clear of them as you can." This seemed like excellent advice in this new setting, albeit difficult to achieve.

Her other related thought was around what she called "mindless" activity: to keep myself quietly, happily occupied, cooking, walking, watching old movies on TV, doing embroidery, anything which stopped me from dwelling too much on these new feelings, yet did not put me into the position of actually having to repress them again.

It seemed it was being suggested I do three things: allow the feelings time and space in which to surface, live in such a way that they did not become overwhelming, and slowly integrate them into the fabric of my life. When later, on return to Australia, I came across the word "idle" in the sense of being ready and waiting to move at the appropriate time, I realised I had been idling in Sweden. I had slowed the pace of my life and

---

29 See *Owning and Honouring*, p. 70

left time and space for my feelings to come up. Since my conscious mind was quieter, not as jam-packed with ideas, theories and explanations as had previously been the case, I allowed myself time to develop and broaden contact with my unconscious, and simultaneously kept myself content with quietly creative activities.

I took up patchwork at this time, something else I had long wanted to do, but for which there had never been time in my pressured work and family-oriented life in Canberra. The Stockholm house was large so I converted a spare bedroom into my quilting room. There with a beautiful view over the Baltic Sea. I spent many mornings planning, cutting and stitching a farmyard quilt for Samantha, my eldest grandchild. I loved the metaphor in the quilting: I was cutting up former dresses — my past — and stitching them into something quite new and beautiful. If I cut or stitched carelessly the pieces would not fit; I would have to re-do it. Was the quilt making showing me what I was doing in my unconscious travels? I imagine so.

The normal life of a diplomat on an overseas posting also provided its own rhythm and sense of order. This was a life I had lived for many years and with which I was very familiar. In the turbulence of my personal life in Sweden it was comforting to have the well-known ritual of attending the receptions and dinners of others and organising those Ian wanted to offer in his turn. We had visitors from Australia to stay in the house, and travelled officially in Sweden, and in Norway and Finland where Ian was also Ambassador.

And so gradually, I found in my own life the stability I needed. Norma, the wife of the Canadian Ambassador, became a close and trusted friend. Having previously done training for voluntary work in a hospice, she had her own experiences of surfacing feelings. Moreover, she shared the preoccupations of my current life, be it a visiting Foreign Minister, the need for extra waiters, an unsettled child at home, or my need to buy the necessary out-door clothes for a Stockholm winter. Together we walked our dogs and talked both in my woods and hers: I felt soothed and steadied.

Slowly my feelings surfaced, slowly I learnt to handle them, integrate them into my existing adult life, gradually I began to feel a different person, one who understood herself, could relate to herself. Walking in the woods...[30]

[30] It seems clear that my situation in Stockholm was unusual in that my feelings came unexpectedly quickly, I was attempting to complete the training in the minimum time recommended and I had few of the normal peer support networks. Most of my fellow trainees and most of the trainees in the Australian training program have continued full or part time work, had normal family relationships and dealt with their new-found feelings all at the same time.

Sharing
Owning and Honouring

"*We'll start with sharing this morning,*" was a statement I heard with misgivings many times during my training. Since this was classic experiential teaching, there was never any explanation of the purpose of sharing. We were just asked to share; sometimes in the big group — all fifty-five of us — sometimes in smaller groups of ten or so. In the big group a sharing session could last two hours or more, the chairs were upright and hard, and I sometimes had problems following the nuances of what was being said despite the presence of translators. I found much of this long and tedious. Although I shared like the good girl I was, I doubt I ever really grasped the importance of sharing feelings in those sessions. At most I felt myself touched by what was said by others — feelings expressed by others released feelings in me; and at times I could see projections involved[31] — participants were projecting feelings around mothers, for example, on some of the women teachers.

Recently, however, some years later, in an Australian intensive that I was attending as an assistant, a fundamental issue arose during a sharing: for whatever unknown reason participant A had not shared during the week; participant B was uneasy at the absence of her sharing. There was a lack of harmony, an exchange of views — "you should share," "you shouldn't expect me to share." It was clear both had problems around the expression or non-expression of feelings: each was playing out her

[31] I am here using the word projection in a general meaning, as for instance in the Macquarie Dictionary: "...that tendency to attribute to another person, or to the environment, what is actually within oneself." Readers interested in some of the psychological technicalities of the concept of projecting are referred to Edward C. Whitmont, *The Symbolic Quest*, Princeton University Press, Princeton, 1978, pp. 60-63.

problem in the intensive, each expecting the other to meet her emotional needs.[32]

As I listened that morning, I suddenly understood one critically important aspect of sharing in my Rosen training. Not only did we learn to receive and give sessions, but we were also being asked to learn to express and handle our surfacing feelings with others in a group setting. In effect we were taking the first difficult steps in applying the knowledge we were gaining about ourselves to the living of our lives. Most participants are initially vulnerable, uncertain, hesitant. An undercurrent runs through the room: Dare I say...? Dare I show...? What will happen if...?

So sharing as I saw years later becomes the place where participants use the presence and personalities of each other, the teachers and assistants, combined with all the different feelings and situations in the room, to help them feel, understand, disentangle and express their own new-found feelings. Hitherto consciously unknown, these feelings have been seen largely in the actions of others, as is the way with the unknown contents of the unconscious. A sharing can become almost theatre-like as participants play out the feelings that are surfacing from their unconscious — an authoritative or loving parent projected on one of the teachers, a sibling on one of the participants, a childhood incident on the general situation in the room.

In such a situation, it is of paramount importance that participants own, take responsibility for, their own feelings. We need practice in spotting projections, recognising the re-enactment, the power of the childhood incident, and attempting to move forward. I needed to realise, for example, the projection that, when feeling like a powerless child facing an apparently omnipotent parent, in reality I am an adult participant, with my own power to make choices, facing a teacher with limited authority.

However, also required for the emotional safety of the group in an intensive is a recognition of the need to honour the feelings of others. If I honour a feeling, I attempt to stay free, cool, not allowing myself to become entangled in the projections of others, while at the same time

[32] Any reader present during the exchange in that intensive, will understand that I have simplified and slightly exaggerated the situation the better to make my point.

I try to recognise their right to their feelings. Notice I said attempt! This is difficult at the beginning. Yet if everyone owns their feelings and honours the feelings of others they will learn to recognise this and recover more quickly from unconscious projections.

Thus in that Australian intensive, step one for participant B was to reclaim her projection and own her own feelings, "For reasons I don't yet understand it is important to me that other people share their feelings"; and for participant A to own her feelings and to honour the feelings of others, "I understand that it is important for you that I share, but for reasons I don't understand it is really difficult for me at the moment." This way there is honesty and integrity over feelings, and the possibility that each may integrate her feelings and move towards transformation, simultaneously allowing another to do the same.

How does this differ from the behaviour of the stereotype yuppies in TV comedies who, having counselling or therapy, talk repeatedly, seemingly endlessly, of their "issues"? Surely this is not what is meant by owning feelings. What is happening here? Seemingly, these comedy caricatures have built the issues around the unearthed incidents into their adult identities. They become people with abandonment issues, authority issues, trust issues: people who, asserting they have these problems, choose not to take responsibility for, not to own, their own feelings. Instead, choosing to play the victim, "I have an authority issue, look what happened to poor little me," they burden others with their feelings. Similarly, so engrossed are they with their own problems, they rarely think to honour the feelings of others. Their relationships are usually awkward, unsatisfactory, as others are forced to manoeuvre around them.

It is easy to fall into this trap, I know I do it from time to time, particularly when the material from the past first surfaces. Then another choice needs to be made: victim or freed-man, freed-woman; do I stay a victim of my past or do I choose to move beyond it, to use the pain of the past to help illuminate the future.

While writing this piece I have been re-reading the biography of Dorothy Ross, the Headmistress of the large Anglican girls school

I attended in Melbourne in the 1940s. One of Australia's leading educationists at that time, she introduced individual timetabling for secondary students (to permit individual development) and the management of much of the everyday affairs of the school by a Council of Councillors (prefects) elected by staff and students. Her stated intention was to provide an environment in which to encourage the unique potential of each student, while at the same time developing in each a sense of their responsibility to the community as a whole.

Owning and honouring, owning our own feelings, our potential, concurrently honouring the feelings, the potential of others, learning to be responsible citizens in the world of expressing feelings, it has taken many years but at long last I understand, this is what the sharing in an intensive is all about, owning and honouring...

This Above All to Thine Own Self Be True

Dear Friend,

Hamlet, isn't it, "this above all to thine own self be true" — being true to oneself, and hence not being false to any man. Over the years, I have wondered about these words: what did they mean? I saw them first in terms of personal integrity, personal honesty. If I was "true" to myself I would be true to others — I didn't lie, scheme, manipulate, knife in the back, advance my own cause at the expense of others. That form of "trueness" has always had a place in my heart. My parents were people of integrity; Ian is, as am I and my children. So it is safe for me to practise Rosen Bodywork; I can be trusted not to manipulate my clients.

This is outward looking, though, it involves my being true to others. What I am now trying to understand are the ramifications of being true to myself. It seems axiomatic that to be true to myself, I must know myself. As I meditated and commenced my Rosen training unconscious feelings began to surface. When I started to reflect on judging, I saw I had not been judging myself in the true meaning of that word — assessing, valuing and discriminating. Rather I had been unconsciously condemning myself out of hand: I never gave myself a chance, I was always wrong, convicted before my defence counsel had even opened his mouth.[33] "Off with her head," as the Queen of Heart's says in Alice in Wonderland.

Then my mind made a leap; to condemn myself out of hand in this way is to reject myself. Ah, now I am approaching familiar territory: fear of rejection by others surfaced early in my Rosen Method training as another of the strong feelings buried in my unconscious. This, then, is a classic case of projection: to fear the rejection of others, when in fact

[33] See *Judge Jeffries — Hanging Judge*, p. 94

unconsciously, I am busily rejecting myself. Now I see where I have been — so busy rejecting myself, condemning myself, that I didn't even know what myself was on about. I hardly knew myself at all.

If I pause and ask my self what am I about, what is the one word in the English language that grabs me; the response, the word that floats up from my unconscious, is love. If unconsciously, judging/condemning has been one essential in my life, love has been another. I want to offer it, to receive it, live it, as it were. What sort of a cross do I make for myself if, on the one hand I want love, and on the other, I am forever judging or condemning myself. The answer that comes is not all that attractive, it may be, probably is, condemnatory. It seems that unconsciously I may be driven to appease.

When we were kids older girls and bullying boys used to give what were called "burns". They twisted your arm until it "burnt", until they reduced you to tears. We use the expression "to twist someone's arm", to force them to do something we want them to do regardless of their own wishes. And they do it, they appease us; they don't want the sore arm. This is a form of abuse.

The brother of a close school friend, four years older than both of us, used to derive great pleasure from twisting my arm; I hated it. Over the years I have seen much abuse, both my own and that of many of my clients. Ingrid was later to say it was reflecting to me something about myself.[34] So it was, of course. I, Judith, unconsciously manoeuvring, dancing around, seeking love, fearing condemnation, was rarely true to myself. I didn't even understand the self to whom I was required to be true. I never stopped to find out; I was too busy condemning, rejecting, abusing myself — albeit all of it quite unconsciously.

So what do I mean, if I write that henceforth I will try to be true to myself? An idea, a word comes up, honouring, to honour one's feelings, to honour oneself. Does that take me further forward or have I simply used one word instead of six?

On reflection I think the idea of honouring myself takes me further. In Jungian terms to honour oneself means to treat oneself and one's

---

[34] See *The Mirror of Life*, p. 153

feelings with respect, care and dignity. If I allow the feelings involved in any situation to come to fruition and play themselves out as constructively as possible, then I am honouring my feelings and also the feelings of others. If feelings are honoured and not repressed, there will be fewer projections. And, if there are no projections in a relationship, then at one and the same time I am being true to myself by honouring (allowing) my own feelings, and also being true to others by not dumping on them all my own projections and allowing them their own feelings.

It's complex, isn't it? I am not sure I have done it justice. All I know for sure and that seems so clear, is that suddenly being true to myself and honouring feelings have become a central part of my being.

What happens if I go one step further and try to be true to My Self, the Divine, the Life Force, God, whatever word I use? Now, all of a sudden, Friend, I see it. It is so obvious, so stunningly simple it quite takes my breath away. Once I know myself, once I allow myself to honour myself and my feelings, no manoeuvrings, no repressions, then I am being true to my self. In similar vein, if I allow those people with whom I am in contact the same freedom, then I am permitting them to be free to themselves. Then, as I see it, I am operating in Divine Mode; I am that small part of the Divine which is Judith, just exactly as she is, with all of her seen, none of her repressed and none of her projected on to others. That way, also, she permits everyone else to be in Divine Mode.

PART III

Lost Innocence

If you bring forth
what is within you,
what you bring forth
will save you.

If you do not
bring forth
what is within you,
what you do not
bring forth
will destroy you.

Jesus
The Gospel of Thomas
Gnostic Gospels

"What's Happening, Judith?"

Ingrid is lovely. We first met in Stockholm in a group of Rosen people having coffee; she was a certified Rosen practitioner and I was in the second year of my Rosen training. At that time my conscious mind registered curly grey hair, steady grey-green eyes, a lovely speaking voice and a Swedish woman with excellent spoken English. Later my intuition said, "You should have some of the twenty-five private, personal Rosen sessions required in the final year of your training from Ingrid."

When I went for my first session, I felt as if I had come home. There was Ingrid, warm and welcoming in the front hall; I seemed to be looking at myself. I glanced around, books, Persian rugs on polished floors, gleaming copper, bowls of flowers. It could have been one of my favourite rooms in any of the twenty houses I had lived in during my diplomatic rambling. My heart sang. I felt safe, in out of the cold of the last two years as the only non-Swedish speaker in the Rosen training. Here it seemed was a guide, a trusty travelling companion with whom I would be able to explore the depths of my unconscious. It was a lovely meeting.

If I ask myself what is my abiding memory of those early Rosen sessions with Ingrid, for in all there were about twenty of them, the word that comes immediately is wonder — the wonder of it. I arrive, we talk a little of how I have been since my last session, if there is anywhere I would like her to work, any part of my body that feels tense or painful. Then I lie face down on her massage table dressed only in my knickers and covered with a blanket. She puts her hands on my body; she has lovely hands, firm and sure, yet sensitive and delicate. Slowly she begins to touch my body working with the muscle tension, quietly, silently at first. Gradually I begin to feel "movement" within — flutters of feelings, fragments of facts — which build slowly into a memory, an insight. When she speaks, her voice is quiet and interested. I know she is really listening to me, which of itself is a lovely thought. "What's happening, Judith," she asks, "what's this about?"

So quietly and gradually, without any trauma or drama, I enter the world of my unconscious — a world initially of repressed childhood memories and their associated feelings. Later as our sessions deepened, a world of undreamt beauty as I discovered feelings of joy, of creativity, of unconditional love, of freedom.[35]

Superficially my session could have been seen to resemble a conventional massage session where only rarely is contact made with the unconscious. So how does the contact in a Rosen session come about? Our mutual focussed intention to listen to the wisdom of my body seems to be the key, for it is this that has brought us together. Her training as a Rosen practitioner and my openness to the process make it possible.

The resemblance to traditional massage is more apparent than real. Ingrid's hands move slowly, sometimes hardly at all, however, they touch deeply. She doesn't talk very much, yet when she does, she talks specifically to my body quietly, slowly — what's happening here Judith? She uses very simple phrases almost as if talking to a child. As she is, of course, for she is talking to my unconscious and words are not its medium of first choice. As I reply I notice my own voice. The timbre has changed; it is slower, deeper. Sometimes I have no idea before I speak what it is I am going to say: words just float up from another part of me, from my unconscious. It is for this reason I use the words "I heard myself say", to describe what happens.

---

[35] See the sessions described in Part IV, *Digging for Joy*, p. 127

As Ingrid worked a picture would gradually build up. In the session where I first experienced my own birth, for example, as she began to work the crown of my head it began to tingle and prickle. Gradually the imagery and feelings I describe in *Birthday* began to surface.[36] Sometimes the image builds quickly, at others it comes more slowly: I see a house I know I have lived in, a room I recognise, people I remember and then suddenly there is a sequence of events of which I have no current conscious recollection. Yet it is relatively easy for me to accept them for they float up in a setting I recognise.

My one control in all of this is to stop the session at any time I choose. I know I can simply open my eyes and sit up. I did this once only when having the session I have described in *The Sleep-Out*[37] with its memories of previously unknown childhood sexual abuse. Even then I did not put an end to the session, rather I paused to talk consciously to Ingrid.

Inevitably some of these recollected memories are painful, that was why I repressed them as a child. In particularly difficult sessions I developed the technique of "moving out" of my body as it were, imagining, "seeing" myself standing beside the table watching myself have that session. "Yes there I am on the table, yes these memories are painful, but if I stand as if watching myself having them, the pain is less intense." At other times I tried to think of memories of a painful situation in general rather than particular terms: not my pain on being unable to breast-feed my first child, rather the pain of any mother in that situation. Both these visualisations seemed to help by putting a space between me and my sensation of pain.

Was I afraid before or during those early sessions? It seems quite probable, since my first session with Ake had shown that fear of the unknown was one of the most powerful of my hitherto unconscious feelings.[38] As I write of fear, I see myself on Ingrid's table. "There's a closed door in front of me," I hear myself say, "I am not sure I want to open it." And then her quiet voice, "You're quite safe," she says, "let your curiosity carry you through, it's a good feeling." Curiosity, yes she was right, it is a good feeling, and I know I am innately curious, so perhaps my curiosity

---

36 See *Birthday*, p. 110

37 See *The Sleep-Out*, p. 92

38 See *A Leap in the Dark*, p. 35

carried me beyond what fear I might have had. That and my trust in Ingrid: for it seemed as if every cell in my body was telling me that with her I was quite safe.

I was usually on her massage table for about fifty to sixty minutes — the length of a classic Rosen session. As the session came to an end, I would normally be lying on my back and she would ask if there was anything else I wanted to mention. Sometimes a word or phrase would float up illuminating the whole of the session; sometimes not. Then she would leave me to rest quietly on the table while she left the room. If a session, such as The Sleep-Out, had brought really tough memories, she might offer me a cup of tea before I left and suggest that I contact her if I had any problems before my next session.

Our Rosen training was emphatic that neither as clients nor as practitioners did we discuss the content of a session immediately it finished. The purpose of the session is to make contact with feelings in the unconscious. The impact of those feelings is lost if we immediately begin to dissect, analyse, and generally put them under the microscope of our conscious minds. Since Ingrid also practised as a therapist, she and I discussed the handling and integration of my surfacing feelings at other times.[39]

In all I saw Ingrid with varying degrees of regularity for about twelve months. After my session, I would go quietly home, collect Sabina and go for one of my "meditation" walks. In my case an incident usually appeared in its entirety in one session, only very occasionally would I see any further imagery. However, over the next few days or weeks I would make contact with other feelings related to what had come up in my session. The whole process was upsetting, no doubt about that. I cried a good deal and, experiencing those previously repressed feelings became angry, felt despairing, powerless and abandoned. I relieved myself of much of the upheaval of those feelings by walking Sabina, talking to Ian and writing letters to my dear friend. Any other spare time away from my diplomatic life, I filled with Amy's mindless activity — working at my patchwork quilt, cooking and watching old movies on satellite television.

---

[39] Rosen practitioners who are not trained therapists, refer clients who have made contact with deeply disturbing feelings to a counsellor or therapist. Sometimes a client takes a break from bodywork while the destabilising feelings are integrated, sometimes the verbal therapy and bodywork continue in tandem.

As the weeks turned to months I slowly began to disentangle myself from the painful immediacy of those recovered feelings and to glean an understanding of the impact on my psyche of those early childhood incidents. To see what had happened that caused me to develop into the woman I then was in the 1980s. That process, it appeared, was threefold. First, I had to see what had actually happened, to make contact with a repressed incident and its associated feelings, usually in a Rosen session. Secondly, I had to feel, to actually live, re-experience in another setting that incident and those feelings so that I had a living knowledge of them and how they might be affecting me in my daily life all those years later.[40] Finally, I began to see a glimmer of my own psychological profile. This whole process took time, weeks, months and, in the case of the most deeply ingrained feelings, even years.

And so we come to those childhood incidents I recollected in the sessions I had during my Rosen training. I have written of these incidents with only a little context or explanation for that is how they occurred. The unconscious, the wisdom of the body, has its own unknown timetable; "stuff", to use the in-house jargon, just comes up, unexpectedly and quite disconcertingly at times. Letters to my dear friend contain glimpses of the many feelings I was experiencing. Since feelings flow, merge, entangle and disentangle as they live and grow, their implications are better understood with hindsight. I have therefore chosen to collect the psychological implications of those feelings, as I came to understand them, together at the end of this part in the tale called *Through a Glass Darkly*.[41]

40 See *The Mirror of Life*, p. 153

41 See *Through a Glass Darkly*, p. 116

Point Leo
Land of Opposites

When I was a small child, in the late 1930s, we used to have family summer holidays at Point Leo — a small, yet beautiful beach about eighty kilometres south east of Melbourne. In those days the entire summer population consisted of those living at the two beach cottages, the twelve or so guests at the boarding house, and some campers: all of us keen surfers. There was no phone, no shop, no tennis, golf or bowls. I knew it only as a beautiful beach with its white, squeaky-clean sand, where I used to walk and play. That playing was important. I was an only child, suddenly there were built-in family play-mates: building sandcastles, exploring the unknown and hidden treasures from the depths of the rock-pools with my mother; skipping, running, surfing with my father.

By Australian standards the surf was only average but steady and relatively sure for the slope into the water was gentle and there were no currents and little under-tow. As a five or six year old I revelled in that moving water; I still do. I love the sea, it is one of the great joys of my life, but it is the surf that really has my passion. I can't remember ever learning to swim. In my first memories I see myself on a small rectangular rubber raft, hanging on for dear life as a wave carries me through the swirling, boiling water to the safety of the water's edge.

I had to learn to respect the surf. Twice I was badly dumped: once as a young child, thrown off my small raft, tossed hither and thither through the swirling water until rescued by an adult friend, and handed back to my father. Later in life, surfing alone with my four young children, I painfully dislocated my right shoulder and had to drag myself back to safety in the shallows.

The guesthouse at Point Leo was tiny: could sleep only eleven people in five bedrooms. As an adult I had no recollection of our family sleeping arrangements, other than hearing a little apprehensively one year that I was now " too big to be sharing with Mummy and Daddy" and was therefore to share a room with Joan, an unknown adult. It came, therefore, as an enormous surprise in one of my early Rosen sessions with Ingrid to see myself lying in the third bed of the only three-bed bedroom.

No longer warm, light, and playfully loving, the atmosphere had changed. Things were happening that, in my sheltered and lovingly protected six year old life I had never ever seen before, never ever dreamt were possible. I lay cowering, shivering in my bed, blankets pulled right up to my neck. It was dark so I could not see where my father was, although it seemed he was in my mother's bed; there were whispers, crying, violence, more angry whispers, and then crying. I shivered and shook and sobbed.

Then my father was in my bed; strong arms round me, rough face against mine, petting, soothing, comforting. Yet, he too was, or had been, crying, his face was wet with tears. I felt bewildered, overwhelmed, confused, absolutely out of my depth as my small world rocked and spun.

Where was my mother? I wanted my mother telling me it was all right, that my loving harmonious world was still there. But my mother was unavailable, a sobbing mound under a pile of blankets in another bed. Yes, my father was there with me, but fathers do not cry. I didn't want him crying in my bed; I wanted him to go away, to leave me alone. It was all too much — I just couldn't handle it, cope with it, any of it...

The scene moved, I saw a tremendous thunderstorm at Point Leo, clouds banging over head, lightning flashing, forking across the bay. I wouldn't go to the window, wouldn't watch, hung back frightened and trembling. "Come and sit with me," said one of the other guests, "I'll tell you about it, it's not nearly so frightening if you understand." As I watched that scene unfold, he encircled me in warm, comforting arms and explained the otherwise inexplicable. I felt safe, secure and slowly gained courage to look at the fury of the storm. Nobody explained that storm in the bedroom, though; it thundered destructively for years.

Point Leo, site of the first loss of innocence. Although my conscious memories were of happy family times, my unconscious tells another tale. Never again, at least unconsciously, would I feel so loved, so safe and secure in my warm and harmonious little world. [42]

A few days later during one of our weekly Rosen training classes, I had another related Rosen session from Anna, a woman with whom I had had little previous contact — simply because she was one of those in the class who spoke no English. We asked Ann-Margret to work with us to help with the talking. It was quiet and peaceful at first. Suddenly an acute pain surfaced in my left shoulder and then flashed sharply right across my upper back. Simultaneously I seemed to be enveloped in a dense black cloud. What on earth was this about? The first fleeting feelings were not so much of fear as those of helplessness, powerlessness and ignorance in the presence of great, monstrously great power.

Gradually the blackness settled; took on the shape of a huge hairy monster, or so it seemed, crouched across my shoulders, gripping me with the claws of all four paws, pushing me down on the table, shouting at me, "You're second-rate, not good enough, never will be good enough no matter what you do, just can't cope no matter how you try." The original monkey on the shoulder, perhaps. I moved, writhed, squirmed, heaved trying to break free: it's no easy matter to throw a monkey off your shoulders lying face down on a table. I was struggling and confused. Lisen, the teacher in charge of the class, came to help Anna and Ann-Margret work my back. At last with one huge almighty heave he, whatever, whoever he was, was off, gone.

---

[42] See *The Stigmata: A Branded Little Soul*, p. 97, for a description of a session some years later, in which other aspects of the events at Point Leo surfaced.

The pain moved to my lower back, sharp, penetrating, all pervasive as if someone were putting in a knife. "Your body is old and tired, not young and pretty, why don't you give up?" were the words I heard in my mind and spoke aloud. "Who", asked Lisen, "who is saying all these things to you?" I lay quietly for a minute and then a moment of truth from my body on the table. "Nobody", I replied, "nobody at all, I am saying them to myself, my mind is saying them."

Despair — Confiding in My Friend

Dear Friend,

I wonder if I can write to you this morning, to put words on paper would certainly help to steady me, could even possibly help to clarify for me where I find myself just at the moment. It is a nasty spot, that's for sure, and one that has previously been completely unknown to me.

Yesterday's dawn brought feelings of total despair, not just for any one isolated incident in my life, but for the second-rate, imperfect and inadequate outcome of everything I have ever attempted. I was, it seemed, quite simply just never good enough. These feelings that were crawling out of every cell in my body, every pore of my skin, with ever increasing intensity (nasty, slimy feelings), were not ones I had previously associated with myself, at least not consciously. Nor, I discovered, were they sharp, noisy, demanding feelings of anger, rage, or frustration at being wrongly judged, to which I was accustomed. Rather I felt cold, absolutely lifeless; I was as if dead, stunned by the hopelessness of it all. It seemed clear that despite all my endeavours I had not been, am not, and never will be good enough. There seemed nothing more to be said or done. I could only pray for a spot of Grace to move me on from this nasty wayside halt.

You, Dear Friend, if you could respond, would be telling me robustly that such feelings are nonsense and I must know it, as another close friend once did when I was working at the Law Faculty. Then I was overborne with feelings of inadequacy as I struggled to write an article for a legal journal on a difficult, challenging topic. Ultimately, though, I now realise, all that bracing and comforting from others is transient, of no lasting effect. Ultimately, it seems, I have to find feelings of my own value from somewhere within myself. Only then will those feelings be stable and permanent; only then will I be able to integrate them and move forward. Say a prayer for me, Friend tis a miserable little wayside halt I have found lately and any feelings of my own value seem as far away as the moon.

Let's hope I can move on soon...

The Sleep-Out
The Cold

The sleep-out, my space in the house of my early childhood, was an area of the side verandah, enclosed to about six feet with canvas covered wooden trellis, above which were hessian curtains on big rings; no bricks and mortar, no solid wood, no glass, a cold, cold unprotected place. I had no idea, until I started my Rosen sessions, how much I hated that space. The house was old, the keys lost, so even worse than the cold, was the possibility that, if the only door was accidentally shut, I could be locked outside and unable to reach the warmth and light inside. Suddenly in one session with Ingrid I saw myself there: alone, afraid and out in the cold.

I was lying face down on Ingrid's table. As she was working my feet, a picture began to develop: Tom, an elderly, lonely neighbour was doing things that most definitely should not have been done. For the only time in my life I stopped the session, leant up on my elbows, "Can you see what I can see?" I asked. Ingrid, well trained and wily, asked in reply, "What can you see?" "I can hardly believe what I can see," I responded. I paused for a minute, then lay down again; she worked quietly on.

The film wound on frame by frame: Tom was partially unclothed, his woollen long-johns hanging over the bed head. I know he used to wear those, for I remember that I had seen them on his clothes line. As the session progressed there was warmth and closeness. At first it appeared I was happily playful to be so close.

Then drama, the scene changes: I am underneath him, squashed and trapped, I am wriggling and squirming, trying to make space, air for myself. In the confusion I get a splash of semen and bite him. In great pain he lashes out, clips me over the right ear with something cold and hard and, "Brazen little hussy!" he shouts, as he grabs his clothes, re-dresses, and storms off. I watch as he goes through the door: shoulders drooped, head down, he passes out of sight.

Ingrid worked quietly on; "Did you tell anyone?" she asked. We waited to see what my unconscious had to say. "Yes," I replied after awhile, "I can see myself sitting on my mother's lap, on the old sofa in the sitting room, I have my arms round her neck; I am whispering to her what happened, what Tom did to me." "And...?" she asked, I waited for a bit, watching the scene, "My mother's saying don't be silly, darling, Tom wouldn't do a thing like that", I reported. Oh, ho, wouldn't he just, some fifty odd years later we both knew better.

Out in the cold for sure now: not only the physical cold of the sleep-out, but the psychological cold of confusion and self-mistrust. Had I mistaken what Tom wanted me to do? Am I right, or have I misunderstood what someone wants me to do? And even more confusing, when someone contradicts me about what I think to be the case, am I incorrect after all? Ultimately, with the end of World War II, the era of the sleep-out came to an end; I had a warm sunny bedroom of my own from which I was not dislodged by visitors. However, the confusion, hesitation, uncertainty and self-mistrust brought about by this incident were to bedevil me for decades.[43]

[43] See *The Stigmata*, p. 97 for further insights into the sleepout incident.

Judge Jeffries — Hanging Judge[44]

Hello Friend,

Greetings from a beautiful beach, always favourite haunts of mine over the years. For some reason I always feel at peace on a beach, even if superficially my life does not appear to be in such good shape. Amy used to say they were my places of "healing", even if I was unaware of the fact.

Healing, so many facets to that jewel. And which one comes to mind today? Relief from that merciless, seemingly eternal inner voice that condemns me, says that I am inadequate, not good enough, never OK, despite my ceaseless strivings. Over the years there have been countless sagas on this theme and some previous encounters with this judge. Recently a small alleviation has begun; it is like a sparkling refreshing drink on a summer's day — relief at long last.

Yesterday I pottered up the main street here looking for a new bathing suit. I felt no pleasure at the prospect. Over the last three or four months I have gained four or five kilos in weight; all my clothes are too tight at the waist. I was dreading a scene where the clothes I like and want to buy won't fit me, and I am left feeling fat, unloved and having to make do with my second and, to my mind, unsatisfactory, choices.

I wandered into a shop. To my surprise, I found a range of bathing suits that not only fitted me comfortably, but also looked good. It was not a question of making do with this when I wanted that, but which one of two or three I would select. I talked to the owner, a pleasant helpful woman, of my perception of my weight problems, my figure. She gave me her perception, which was quite, different. We isolated two for a final choice. "Do you want to look smart or pretty?" she asked.

---

[44] Judge Jeffries (1645-1689) was a prosecutor, judge and ultimately, in 1683, Lord Chief Justice of England. As a prosecutor he was notorious for bullying and savagely ridiculing defendants; as a judge he had a reputation for the ferocity and severity of his sentences sending many hundreds into slavery in American colonies and ordering the execution of hundreds more. His behaviour all those centuries ago, led to the coining of the phrase, Hanging Judge, for any mercilessly severe judge.

"Pretty," came my immediate answer. So I walked out with a brand new bathing suit that showed off my sleek bum, concealed my slightly thickening middle, all in stunning shades of pink and mauve, *and* feeling a million dollars.

See the gift I was offered by an unknown shop owner: I could be either pretty or smart. "Oh," I replied, "I am not the gold chain, gold bracelet, red painted nails type. I will be pretty." Suddenly I turned new eyes on my other clothes. It's true, I am not smart, I used to aspire to that, not any longer. That word I now associate with a certain hardness, an absence of the true feminine, and in most cases, with the not so old. As I looked at my clothes with my new eyes I saw that many of them, if not smart, were pretty: soft colours, good designs looking good on me. Maybe one can't be smart at nearly sixty, but one can still look pretty.

So what's all this about? A simple action, a woman goes shopping, happens all the time! And when she does she is up against an arbitrary and inflexible measuring stick, current fashion and the shop owner's interpretation thereof. A twentieth century version of a hanging judge; fit this standard or you fail — have no clothes! It is a strong serene woman who comes home from such an encounter purring with satisfaction. One who is very happy in her own body. And that has not been me, certainly not these last few months.

As I strolled back in the sun to our unit by the sea I saw where I had been. I have not been well. Tired almost to death, battling the "I can't cope" syndrome, my body has seen fit to pile on the weight. Then, since New Year, I have had continuing problems with my right ear bringing dizziness, nausea and loss of hearing. I have felt weak, breathless and very conscious of an approaching birthday. So watch my unconscious Judge at work: I'm fat, not at all attractive, hard of hearing and *old* (for in my book at that time I know not why, approaching sixty is old, finished, passed it). See that Hanging Judge, he's been there all summer, beavering away in my unconscious, insidiously poisoning my decision to have some weeks of rest with his sneaky snide messages of weakness, inadequacy and advancing age.

Somehow that shop owner had shut the Judge up, given me some respite, helped me to another perception of myself. Jolted me too into remembering, seeing clearly where I am: not weak, inadequate, old, deaf, past it; but *resting*, dear God, *resting*, can I never hear that word; *resting* after the vicissitudes of the last couple of years. I alone know what they have cost me. You have a pretty fair idea, so do Ingrid and Amy; but the true balance sheet is known to me alone. If I can shut the Judge up, just for a moment I can hear a voice say "You are doing well, very well, it's a long tough haul, effectively a self-analysis; much of it alone. Give yourself a break, for God's sake, have a rest, just let yourself be."

Helping a friend move house last weekend, tired and ragged, I finally flew at two constantly needling small children. "Oh be quiet!" I shouted, "if you can't be quiet, just go away and leave us in peace." And so off they went and peace descended — the relief.

However, all the literature says that I can't shout at the figures in my unconscious and send them away. Ultimately I have to come to terms with them, integrate them into my full personality. Only then do I become whole, without repressions and without the danger of projections.

A place without condemnatory judges, it sounds like quiet magic. A place where I am no longer judged, no longer judge myself, condemn myself so rigorously; a place, now perhaps not so far off, where *I* listen to *myself*; where I decide, after review of *all* relevant facts whether I am tired, not tired, justified, not justified; whether I am inadequate, old, fat, past it, or just tired, unwell, needing rest. No external community standards, no unconscious needling, no projection on others. Only my own still small voice, no other.

Quite a tall order, Friend. Can I manage? I wonder. Time alone will tell.

The Stigmata
A Branded Little Soul

S*everal years later* the Point Leo and sleep-out incidents surfaced again. One afternoon in March 1995, after Ian and I had left Sweden and returned to live in Australia, I answered the phone and heard a voice say, "Hullo, Judith, it's Jan from Sweden": a voice I had not heard in years; a voice I knew, liked and trusted. He was coming to Australia in October, he said, to be best man at his brother's wedding; was there sufficient interest in Rosen Bodywork for him to give some Introductory Workshops, with the possibility of starting an Australia based Rosen practitioner training program.

And so the wife of the one time Ambassador (itself a busy unpaid public relations job), the former university lecturer, the small time Rosen practitioner, entered a new world: that of the entrepreneur, the business-woman, the promoter who speaks publicly to both press and radio, who organises brochures, conference venues, catering. Similar to the organisation of diplomatic functions? Possibly. It did not feel so at the time. In diplomatic functions you have a list of invitees, of which experience tells a known percentage will probably accept. Here the crux of the matter was that I had no list and no idea how many, if any, people would be attracted. I found those two weeks prior to the workshops busy and intense, and the preceding two months some of the most pressured I remember.

Finally we held two workshops in October from which emerged a small enthusiastic group of people interested in training as possible Rosen practitioners. Jan, who had been one of the pioneers in the Rosen practitioner training program for the then USSR, was brim-full of enthusiasm and ideas. "Isn't it wonderfully coincidental," he said, "Annika," another Swedish Senior Rosen teacher, "will be in Australia on holiday in January 1996, she can conduct another Introductory Workshop. Then our training program will be really under way." But he was leaving, off to his brother's wedding, and then back to Sweden. I, on the other hand, exhausted and burnt out with the strain of his visit and lifting this program off the ground, would be left to do it all again alone in twelve short weeks. Tears came, "I can't do it, I can't manage, I just can't cope...," I murmured.

And so Jan gave me my Rosen session. As he put his hands on my back, the tears trickled again. Oh the relief to have some understanding professional Rosen support after four long years as the only accredited Rosen practitioner in Australia. Ian, my family and my close friends had been wonderfully supportive, offering sound common-sense, business acumen, contacts and a shoulder to cry on; but none had professional knowledge of Rosen Bodywork, that pioneering burden I had carried alone.

I asked Jan to work my right buttock and hip, they had been painful for weeks. First, surprisingly, a new incident. After nearly seven years of bodywork, I thought I had unearthed all the child-hood nasties; but no, here was at least one more. There I was in a house I knew well, playing hide-and-seek with a close childhood friend. I was hiding under the bed when her older brother found me. Pulling me out by one leg, he tickled me viciously, mercilessly. Finally, all but annihilated and sobbing hysterically, I wet my pants. At that he jeered and ridiculed me even more. "Dirty little cry-baby, dirty little cry-baby," he sneered as he left the room.

Jan worked quietly on, always on the right hip/buttock. Tom and the sleep-out surfaced again. One very clear insight here, one I had previously suspected but not confirmed from my body. This time it was clear that when I bit him, whatever my unconscious may have had in mind, consciously I imagined I was doing what he wanted. Never in my wildest dreams could I have dreamt what ensued: the violence, the confusion and the shattering of a precious friendship.

Jan rolled me on my back and, rotating my hip slowly outward, continued to work my hip/ buttock. "Another incident is floating up," I said, " Another man?" he asked, " Yes, my father." The Point Leo incident came again, seemed almost to sing out of the pain in my hip: the images built up. There was more detail this time, more insights. A young couple, my mother and father, in love, on holiday. Although after the death of their baby son in 1935, my mother had been warned she should never become pregnant again, she later did so and was given an illegal (in 1936) abortion by her doctor. So fear of pregnancy and its consequences for her — death — were very real for both my parents, in particular for my mother. My father is really aroused: he knows he shouldn't insist, he knows the risks, he doesn't want his wife to die, but he can't help himself. There is the nasty violent scene I had already seen.[45]

Previously I had pondered the depth of feelings apparently aroused in me as a spectator. As I watched the scene again with Jan I saw further. My father had come into my bed, yes, rocked, soothed, petted me yes; but he was a big man, strong and powerful, he seemed to be all over me. I felt trapped, smothered, powerless, and above all incredibly inadequate.

Jan talked quietly of a stigmata: "It seems," he said, "as if this feeling of 'I just can't cope, leave me alone', is a stigmata for you, so deeply is it branded into your psyche, into your very soul." That felt absolutely right, it has been graven into me, lurking largely unrecognised in my unconscious, but bedevilling me nonetheless over and over again. And here it was again over fifty years later, stirred by the necessity of making the arrangements for another Rosen Introductory Workshop.

Later I discussed this session with Jennifer, my counsellor friend who had become such a source of loving wisdom in my life on my return to Australia. Together we looked at the circumstances in that room at Point Leo as the reason for the depth of my "stigmata, my branding". "Everyone

[45] Point Leo, p. 86

in the room", she said, "was feeling desperately inadequate, unable to cope, wanting to be alone. Your mother feeling she had started it all by refusing sex; your father, in turn feeling he had started it by asking for sex; you in your reactions to what was happening. Every facet of the incident shone with being inadequate, being unsatisfactory, being second-rate, being unable to cope. No wonder you, the smallest and most vulnerable person in the room, had those feelings burnt into your soul."

Bendigo
Dancing Cheek to Cheek

F*red Astaire and Ginger Rogers*, the names conjure up exquisite dancing, wonderful harmoniously moving bodies, catchy, lilting melodies. It is Fred who sings of heaven... of dancing cheek to cheek.

Recently I sat watching my toddling grandson on a terrace; just learning to walk, he had gained the courage to wander off outside alone. He was faraway, dreaming, lost in his own little world, his heaven, cruising quietly, casing his joint as it were, a tentative touch here, a stroke there; would he taste it? Why not! Into his mouth, ugh, not so good. Another touch, a gentle tug; oh this is such fun, he had no idea the world could hold such treasures.

Suddenly I saw myself, a toddler in the garden of the house my parents had occupied in the early 1930s in the large bustling Victorian gold mining town of Bendigo. The garden, it seemed, had been one of my first heavens. I watched myself, a touch, a sniff, into my mouth, a pat, a tug, cruise on quietly, do it all again. What was this?...and this? How I loved these newfound treasures. The sun shone, the bees buzzed, my mother was sitting quietly in her chair, from time to time I took her one of my finds, we explored it together. She turned on the hose, more joy, I splashed the water everywhere; I actually have an old family snapshot of that scene. The chubby toddler holds the hose, the water running out, the happy playful smile.

Bendigo, though, was not only quiet family joy: the joy of my parents, a young couple in love, with their first born daughter. Bendigo brought unexpected tragedy to that young family: changed their lives and mine forever. It was here in Bendigo in 1935 that my brother Tony was born and died three short weeks later of an infection. Here my mother was critically ill with puerperal fever and learned that further children would result in her death. Here my parents' hopes for a large family were dashed. Here I became an only child.

It was here also that my mother was absent for six long weeks as she battled for her life in the hospital. This story was part of our family folklore; I learnt it gradually as I grew up. What I did not know until I did my Rosen training were the feelings of that toddler when she woke to find her mother no longer part of her life, just gone, disappeared without trace; her place taken by a younger woman she did not know, felt uneasy with, and called the Ant.

Lying on a massage table at an early Rosen training session I made contact with that toddler's feelings. We had been sitting in a circle sharing what was going on in our lives (an intrinsic part of Rosen training),[46] a remark sparked something for me, suddenly tears poured down my face. I left the circle, found a blanket and curled up on a table. Soon I was crying uncontrollably, racked with sobs, shivering, rocking to and fro, curled up in a tight little ball, foetus position. "Where is my mother? What has happened to my mother? Why doesn't she come? She always comes when I cry, where is she now?" On and on, round and round, a tiny mouse trapped in her cage of a cot, shivering, peering, frantic, "where is my mother, what has happened to her?"

Ann-Margret came then and sat quietly by the table waiting for the storm to subside. "What is happening, Judith? What is this all about?" "It's my mother, she's gone, left me, abandoned me, rejected me, and I don't know where she is." The garden in Bendigo may have been joy in heaven; this was sheer hell, pain in hell.

The ensuing days brought further flashbacks. Bendigo was rage, tantrums, I didn't want Ant looking after me, didn't like her, didn't trust

---

46 See *Sharing*, p. 70

her. Bendigo was Ant saying it was naughty to go alone into the garden, naughty to get dirty, naughty to play with water and get wet, and oh so very naughty to cry for mummy. Bendigo, so it appeared later in another Rosen session, was Ant saying as she slapped my chubby little leg, that if I was not a good girl mummy wouldn't come back. Where was my sunny blue heaven now? In its place I seemed to have a fog of confusion. My little world was quite upside-down.

Bendigo was also a large, fat, woman, I was later to know as a spinster relative of my father's, saying as she came to see my mother on her return from hospital, "Well, at least you have Judith." What was I, some sort of second class consolation prize? At least you have Judith! I ask you.

A few weeks after these flashbacks, I was in the midst of yet another Rosen intensive. We were to select partners and work on necks and faces, told to work carefully and gently, as these are areas in which many feelings are deeply held. I asked Kajsa to work just behind my right ear: a spot that had been stiff and painful for a couple of weeks.

In minutes I was flooded with image after image of my father and my early childhood. He was in a plum tree, way above the ground, dropping plums down into a sheet I was holding with my mother. He was happy, laughing, carefree, gaily throwing the fruit. I was frozen with terror that he would fall, be killed, leave me alone in this world without my one known trusted safe haven.

She moved to work on my right cheek. At first it brought further painful emotional flashbacks, with physical pain coming and going in blinding flashes. Then I saw my toddler self standing in the cot arms outstretched waiting to be lifted out. I recalled then that about nine months after my father died (in 1964) I had great pain in my right cheek, had finally gone to the doctor, been told it was neuralgia, and given pain-killers. Now it was beginning to appear that all my feelings for my father were held in my right cheek. He must have carried me on his right shoulder. There cheek to cheek was where I felt loved, safe, and totally protected from harm. There rocking, dancing cheek to cheek was my small heaven. When he died it appears that in some curious way the feeling in my right cheek died also. Now some twenty-five years later feeling, movement, dancing were returning. Dancing cheek to cheek...

Duck[47] *— Farewell to My Father*

Dad, dear,

It was February 1962 that you and I said goodbye for the last time as Nick (Ian) and I set out with Jill and Mark[48] on our posting to Phnom Penh, capital of Cambodia — at that time an outpost of civilisation lost in the mists of south-east Asia. We went by ship, and I remember being deeply shaken to find your face wet with tears as we kissed goodbye. And yet that day we neither of us had any idea that this was the ultimate goodbye, that you would die suddenly and unexpectedly as a result of a massive heart attack in 1964 and we would never have the chance to speak again.

I wrote to you last as I recall in mid 1964 suggesting that you and Mum visit us in Phnom Penh for Christmas that year and meet your newest grandchild, due in October. You replied (I have the letter still), that nothing would give you greater pleasure; but that you were still plagued by intuitive fears of an early death and felt therefore that you should stay in Australia, working and saving to ensure that Mum was adequately provided for. Your reply did not surprise me; we had spoken of this before.

Events then overtook both of us: Pip was born in October. A few weeks later I received that dreadful telegram with news of your heart attack. Two weeks later you died — leaving Mum a bereft widow of fifty-nine and me, your young thirty-one year old daughter, stunned and confused. It seems almost unbelievable now, so much have communications improved and travel costs lessened, but at that time it was physically impossible to make a phone call from Phnom Penh to Melbourne, and the cost to us of the airfare to Australia was out of the

[47] Duck was the name by which my father always called me. A little of *The Stigmata: A Branded Little Soul*, p. 97 is repeated here.

[48] Ian and I have four children: Jill born in South Africa, Mark born in Melbourne on our return from Egypt, Penelope (Pip) born in Bangkok while we were posted to Phnom Penh and Bridget born in New Caledonia.

question.[49] So you died and I never spoke to you, never saw you again.

What does it feel like to die young, quickly and unexpectedly, I now wonder? Did you feel bitter or frustrated at so many things left undone; or was there rather a sense of relief, that you could at last put down the burden of life? For the survivors a quick pain-free death looks good: a real blessing in a world of increasingly protracted pain-filled deaths. The survivors, themselves, however, have to handle the anguish of death compounded by the trauma of the unexpected nature of it. Mum found it difficult to recover. She was at first bitter and resentful at being widowed so young; later, increasingly fearful and defensive, as she handled with great courage, the problems of ageing alone.

And me, what was it like for me? At the time I was stunned by grief; my small world shook, but it also had to go on. Pip aged barely six weeks needed care. Mum, in the event, came to Phnom Penh, and my own grieving seemed to have to be put aside — both in order not to upset her, but also to be able to look after her. As the years went by I have noticed in myself a total inability to go to the opera — something you and I used to love to do together — a constant weeping in church, and my own increasing fears that Ian, too, would die young — a fear fuelled by his own intuitions.

Then, three years ago, I started my training in Rosen Bodywork, and one by one the hitherto repressed feelings around your death, and later, the happiness of our life together, began to surface. In my Rosen sessions with Ingrid your death surfaced time and again. There I would be on her table racked by deep sobs and seemingly unable to move forward. Finally one day without giving any reasons she suggested I should write to you. "Go and sit in a very beautiful place, Judith," she said, "take your time, just write to him quietly and lovingly as you would if you were talking to him. Tell him everything, all those things you never spoke of during his life."

So, here I am some twenty-seven years later in my sitting room in Stockholm with its beautiful view over the Baltic. What is it I want to say? First, and in many ways the most important, is the fact that

---

[49] A situation now covered by government entitlement to a compassionate leave airfare.

unconsciously I have never felt "safe" since you died. From all the feelings surrounding Tony's birth and subsequent death, Mum's illness and long absence, it now appears that as a small child I looked to you alone for protection.[50] This unconscious patterning I took into my adult life: you were my rock, my trusted protector in a world I distrusted; a mantle that passed to Ian on your death.

Yet there was conflict in this trust arising from that stormy night at Point Leo. Then, as I have felt it, you moved out of your protective role; first in exposing me to the feelings between you and Mum; secondly, when in trying to comfort me you showed me your own weakness. You were, remember, crying in my bed. What was I, five or maybe six at the time? It seems incredible, unlikely, yet so much of my Rosen work affirms it: on that one stormy night a large part of my own emotional patterning was formed. My feelings of being inadequate, second rate in some way. You were not kind to Mum, do you remember?

Even more bedevilling, my feelings that love necessarily involved dependence. I was crying, you were comforting me; you were crying, I was comforting you. Somehow I grew up feeling that love was a mutual defence pact in which each party undertook to protect and comfort the other around pain. That is true, of course, there is that element of mutual dependence and defence in personal love, but it encompasses so much more, and that I have been slow to learn.

I am sorry this sounds unkind; I don't mean it that way. I just want the story, the whole story, as I see it now, out in the open. You were, I do know, a wonderfully warm, generous and loving father. I have marvelled during my training to hear so many Swedish women talk of their strict, cold, reserved fathers; you were never like that. Our house was warm, loving, filled with light, books, music and insight. People, the lame ducks of this world, came and went; you had a helping hand for them all. You went, too, to dine with the Governor, or to the local pub at Flinders to have a few beers with the fishermen; you mixed easily, naturally with all of them. You had that cool, clear brain, remember?

---

50 See *Bendigo*, p. 101

The ability to see straight to the heart of a problem. People say I have it too.

There was one grief you carried I felt, but rarely saw: the death of Tony, your small son, and the never to be fulfilled longing for further children. I saw that openly once only, when you burst upon me just after Mark's birth. I was on a trolley, going from the labour ward to my room in the hospital. Suddenly you erupted up the stairs, arms full of red flowers, roses, carnations, I can't remember. You were all but weeping, beside yourself with joy, a small grandson, your "son" at last.

It is difficult for me to describe how those feelings of yours affected me as a child. The conscious feelings were vague, insubstantial; as I have worked with my unconscious they have cleared a little. Yet, as I write, there seems a danger of giving too sharp a form to something that was ephemeral. What was it? A hazy feeling that your pride, your love was so deep, so intense it was almost burden-like. I had to struggle to carry it, to live up to it.

Again this is not a criticism, just a statement of the situation as it seemed to me. Here, too, there is another side of the picture. You were so proud of me, you welcomed me fully into your male world (something few fathers did for their daughters in the 1940s and early 1950s). You gave me the freedom to do whatever I wanted with my life, a rare and treasured gift. At the same time you affirmed your love for the woman, the feminine in me your daughter. Do you remember that wonderful, billowing, frothy, lace half petticoat you bought, and gave me one Christmas? How I loved it. I see it still.

Now, as I have come to understand it, this letter is to bring to an end my protracted and initially, largely unacknowledged grieving as a result of your sudden death: the fact that we never spoke, never said good-bye, and that I never had the chance to thank you for your love, your protection, your support in everything I tried to do, your inspiration. Now maybe I will finally be free from the anguish, the pain that your physical presence is no longer with me: in particular freed from that craving for your protection. Now, at fifty-seven, maybe at very long last

I will be able to stand on my own two feet, finally free to move forward as an adult, to feel and use your love, your blessings, your many gifts in the rich and rewarding life that lies ahead.

Bless you,
Duck

First Birth Day

Twelfth of July 1933

"*What do you know of your own birth?*" Ingrid asked during one of my sessions as she worked the top of my head. I lay quiet feeling her touch, firm yet gentle and sure on the crown of my head. What did I know about my own birth? Not a great deal. Family folklore had it that I was so late arriving my mother and father had finally gone to see a funny film, hoping that laughter would spur me on. I mentioned this briefly; it did not seem significant.

As her hands continued to work, my scalp began to tingle and prickle, a picture began to build up.[51] Slowly Ingrid's room slips away. I see a tiny unborn baby in a warm dark space; I recognise her as myself. Although she cannot speak, cannot verbalise or even think thoughts at that time, now in my session looking at the image of that baby, I feel her, feel in myself the feelings of that baby. At first she is almost indescribably beautiful, so alive, afire almost with the joy of living, the joy of life, wriggling, bubbling over with excitement. She seems to know something wonderful is about to happen, that she is about to go on a great adventure; she can't wait for it to begin.

Suddenly she is, I am, enveloped in a thick fog — fear. An overwhelming sensation of fear, seemingly coming from outside, wraps itself around me. Then a series of fleeting almost simultaneous feelings and images: I am in a constricted space — dark, slimy, airless; I'm stuck,

[51] At the time I experienced my own birth with Ingrid my own mother was too frail for me to ask her for details of what had occurred. However, many of my own clients who have experienced aspects of their own births have had confirmation from people who knew the facts at the time.

jammed in, unable to move. And withal there is this fear, this great blanket enveloping, engulfing me, all but paralysing me. Suddenly there is pain, ouch, something cold, hard, unyielding grabs both sides of my head. I am pulled, yanked free from the constrictions and land none too elegantly with gasp and a thump on something hard. Words float up directly from my unconscious. "It was a forceps birth," I hear myself say, "my mother was so frightened she wouldn't, or couldn't push, so I had to be a forceps birth." "Yes," agrees Ingrid, "that's how I saw it also." My body gave a long deep sigh, the "aaaah" of recognition, the aaah that says "so that's what this is all about, that makes so much sense."

Ingrid worked on, I watch myself again, that tiny baby lying on the table: there is a blinding light, people, movement, confusion; yet for one split second, I seem to be alone. "Something must be happening to my mother," I murmur, "everyone seems to be concentrating on her." Tears come as I feel that fleeting second of abandonment. I have finally arrived, yet no one seems to be greeting me. Then I am in my mother's arms, feel the warmth, see her smiling face, the light, the love in her eyes.

The session finished, Ingrid went to sit in her chair; I lay quietly on the table moved to the core of my being. To relive my own birth in this way had been a powerful experience; the feelings involved were intense. And with that aaaah of recognition so much of the emotional patterning of my life fell into place. I knew now that the overwhelming feeling present at my birth was fear: fear, fear and more fear. My mother's fear of childbirth — as it appeared — and later my own fears jammed in the narrow confines of the vagina.

Talking of this session at a later date, Ingrid and I speculated that I had taken on my mother's fear, had it stamped, as it were, onto my own very new and acutely vulnerable unconscious. Certain it is that to this day I hate dark underground places. To be asked to inspect an underground mine, a privilege not normally accorded to women and therefore practically impossible to refuse, was to find myself white, shaky and clammy with fear. A long dark narrow mineshaft, a vagina, the unconscious senses the similarities and sends the related feeling — fear.

Poppy:
Mothers and Daughters, an Archetypal Tangle

When I started my bodywork training in 1988, previously unconscious negative feelings around my mother began to surface: she had abandoned me (at Tony's birth); did not listen to me about Tom ("don't be silly, darling, Tom wouldn't do a thing like that"); and in trying to console me before I was evacuated to the country with my school in WWII, she had totally misled me about how happy I would be, and was therefore, I felt, not to be trusted. At times I was furiously angry with her: "How dare you do that to me?" I roared one day, as I beat up a pillow after a particularly rough Rosen training session. Yet, as I had previously consciously understood it, we had had a happy, relaxed, intimate and loving relationship. I therefore felt puzzled, confused and distinctly uneasy.

It was not simply that I did not like criticising my mother; many people find that difficult. It was also that I too, am a mother, that I had invested a large part of my adult life in trying to be a "good" mother to my four children in the difficult circumstances of diplomatic life, where the inevitable separations place unavoidable strains on families. As I saw it, my life had been an uneasy balancing act as I struggled to keep all family members happy. Thus, I found I couldn't face the thought that my children, if they were to have counselling or therapy now, would also find me lacking as a mother: abandoning them at boarding school; and, when I was responding to Ian's need for my presence, not around at all times to offer them the love, the encouragement and the support to which as my children they presumably felt entitled.

As I did my Rosen training, this constant tension between the daughter in me criticising, and the mother in me fearing to suffer possible criticism, made it almost impossible to see my feelings around my mother with any clarity; inevitably I seemed to become entangled in my own feelings as a mother.

Then I read *Poppy*[52], a novel in the form of a biography of a mother, in which the author/daughter states that until she commenced to write her book, she had never "seen" her mother as a person in her own right, she had only ever seen her as "mother", her mother. The passage leapt off the page and grabbed me, bull's eye.

Suddenly I saw how little I had seen my mother, Mum, as the person she was: Kathleen Wyatt (FitzRoy) born in 1904 and living her own life as daughter, wife, mother and woman in the mid twentieth century. As such she would have had all her own fears, anxieties and personality quirks arising from her childhood and the life she had been obliged to live. Hers had been turbulent times involving the loss of her parent' property in a bushfire, her own father's sudden death, followed by financial struggles and a mortgagee's sale. This in turn was followed by the Depression of the 1930s in which my father (now her husband) struggled to find work for himself and help his bankrupted father and siblings. Last but by no means least were all the upheavals of WWII.

Looked at in this light, she had to go away to have Tony, her second baby, and in 1935, would have been in hospital for at least three weeks even if she had not been ill. She was bound to deny the sexual abuse: no one talked of such things at that time, and in any event, it would never have happened in "nice families" like ours. She felt she had to send me to Marysville during the war, tried to console me the only way she knew how — and to be fair, brought me home as soon as she understood how distressed I was. She had to act this way; for she, my mother, was first and

52 Drusilla Modjeska, *Poppy*, McPhee Gribble, Penguin Books Australia Ltd., 1990.

foremost a woman in those difficult times. Moreover, I had re-lived my birth with Ingrid, seen my mother's face as she held me for the first time, heard the love in her voice as she spoke to me; she loved me, loved me passionately, and did absolutely everything within her limits to give me a good start in life.

That paragraph in *Poppy* showed me where I had been. I had been looking to my mother to be everything one could possibly want from mothers. I had projected the archetype of "the mother", perfect motherhood on the person of my mother and was anticipating my children would do the same to me. *Poppy* showed me I was loving a person, Kathleen Wyatt, who was also a mother, my mother. As a person she was infinitely lovable, quietly courageous, sensitive, full of fun. Yes, the child in me had certainly wanted her to act in other ways; but the adult in me could now be understanding of her difficulties, and trust that my children would have the same understanding for me in similar circumstances.

In December 1993, recovering from a lumpectomy and subsequent radiation therapy for breast cancer, I went first to Washington to meet a new grandson, and then to England to stay with very close friends. On learning I was ill, Ingrid had written from Sweden suggesting the possibility of sessions with a healer, Mathew, who lived not far from Cambridge where I was to spend part of my time.

Mathew worked in a way I had not previously experienced. I was asked to send in advance my medical history and my reasons for wishing to see him. In reply I wrote of the cancer and my need to find balance and emotional equilibrium after the ups and downs of the years of self-analysis that had been the effect of my Rosen training. On arrival, Mathew had my faxed reply; no further details were taken. The sessions were short, thirty minutes only, with little or no talking. The first day he talked quietly of his trips to Australia, his understanding of Australian treatments for cancer. Then playing a CD of beautiful relaxing music, he moved to sit behind me and place his hands at or near different parts of my body. In the two succeeding sessions the full 30 minutes was devoted to music and energy channelling.

The second session brought an image, but more importantly, a feeling of being at one and the same time both daughter and mother. The words to stress here are "at one and the same time". It was as if previously I had always been two people, or at least two aspects of the feminine, a daughter and a mother. There had been constant tension between these two. Now suddenly that fragmentation and its tension went. I saw myself, felt myself, first and foremost as a woman, at times daughter, wife, mother, friend, but basically a woman; with the possibility of freedom from the constraints of all these other roles I had been asked to play, all these archetypal patterns. Judith Nicholson person, woman. Ah, the peace, the possibility of freedom here.

It was some time before I fully understood the impact of reading *Poppy* and that session with Mathew. I saw first that in no longer loving a concept, "Mother", I was growing to love a person, "Mum", and offering to love her unconditionally, freely without expecting any particular response — my old friend, Divine Love.[53] So often we say she is my mother she must do, say, feel such and such. Or alternatively I am her daughter I must do say, feel so and so. This, though, is a human concept of love, the ego-based concept, filled with ideas of obligations, needs, fears and anxieties. At its best it is flawed: at its worst it is a fiend, obsessive, tyrannical and destructive. When it is transformed into Divine Love, though, with its absence of demands and obligations and the ensuing freedom, then there is beauty and peace.

53 See *Beloved…Ah, Beloved*, p. 141

Through a Glass Darkly

D*uring our time in Sweden* we visited Australia more often than we had done on previous postings. Ian's mother was very ill, mine was frail and ultimately died while we were still there. We needed to sell a house we had bought near the Melbourne University as a home away from home for our children. And in our first Swedish winter we had such a longing for Australian sun and sea, that we spent money Ian's mother had given him for Christmas, on a quick trip to see her and to bask in the sun.

During these visits my friends were puzzled when I talked about my Rosen experiences. With few exceptions, they regarded my exploration of my unconscious as eccentric and unnecessary. "Why do you want to stir up all this stuff?" they asked, "why put yourself through this seemingly painful process?" Alternately they retorted, "Me, investigate my unconscious, why on earth would I want to do that?" Yet at this point they would often remark that my bodywork would be great for a spouse, friend or colleague who seemed to have personal problems, or a superior who was treating them unfairly in some way about which they felt powerless. They were alright, they were telling me, but it just so happened they felt someone they knew needed to change how they were behaving and could therefore possibly benefit from Rosen Method Bodywork.

In 1988, on arrival in Sweden with Ian, I too fitted this pattern. I understood little of the unconscious and its workings. I was whingeing about "them", the administrators of the Department of Foreign Affairs and Trade, who in complete denial of the departmental rhetoric about taking the professional interests of spouses into account on postings, had posted Ian to Sweden where it was impossible for me to continue my work as an academic lawyer.

And so I was resentful at what had "been done" to me and wanted change in an area where I felt powerless. It seemed I had two options: I could carry on, consciously feeling irritable, uneasy and powerless and, yes, victimised, a martyr to the circumstances of my life. Or, as my Rosen work was suggesting, I could consider changing myself. With hindsight, it appeared the answer to the question "what was I seeking?", in that first formal Rosen session with Ake[54], was a new outlook on life: one that would carry me contentedly through the next phase of my life. And so it seemed, as was later to be the case with many of my own clients, I was unconsciously drawn to bodywork because I was in physical and emotional pain, stuck or blocked in my life, and searching for I knew not what, just searching...

As my time in Sweden drew to a close I spent my meditation walks seeking to formulate not only the growing psychological awareness of myself that was flowing from my bodywork sessions, but also how that awareness could help me adjust to the changing circumstances of my life. The phrase "through a glass darkly", kept running through my thoughts. I tracked it down in an Epistle from St. Paul to the Corinthians. "For now we see through a glass darkly; but then face to face: now I know in part, then shall I know even as I also am known."

At first I seemed little wiser; yet as I played with the phrase it began to seem wonderfully appropriate. For it was now clear that when I started my bodywork sessions I saw myself through a glass darkly, through a haze of negative feelings, not brought about by any major psychological trauma, but simply by the living of my early family life in the social times of the 1930s and 1940s; at best I knew myself in part only. And now, all

---

[54] See *A Leap in the Dark*, p. 35

these Rosen sessions later, it seems I know, even as I also am known — that is as I now know myself.

See that grimy mirror, the very negative picture I had of myself that emerged as those major childhood incidents surfaced from my unconscious. From the boarding house at Point Leo, this deeply ingrained feeling — Jan's "stigmata" — that I am second-rate, inadequate, unable to cope, never good enough, despite all my efforts. This I now know to be a deeply incapacitating limiting feeling, despite a lifetime, to all outward appearances, of coping quite adequately.

There were further insights from that incident at Point Leo in another later session with Ingrid, "I feel as if my little world is breaking up under my feet," I murmured. "Of course," she replied, "you had never seen anger or violence previously in your loving, harmonious family." This too has had its restricting consequences in later years. Even now, as an apparently confident and competent woman, to be present in the Law Faculty when others argued passionately, to feel family discussions approaching a lack of harmony, to be anywhere in fact in the presence of aggression or quarrels, even emphatic assertion, brings butterflies to my stomach and feelings of near panic. Many years ago Ian said he would have liked to enter politics but felt he was not strong enough and that I would not be able to stand the discord. How right he was; now I can see the roots of that fear in that incident at Point Leo.

Tom in the sleep-out brings forth a major actor in my unconscious drama — my judge. He, for he is male, is the archetypal hanging judge, won't listen, won't hear, merciless and condemnatory: he says to me when I think my actions are right they are wrong. Thus follows a lifetime of unconscious judging, a little voice constantly murmuring "you shouldn't have…"

My mother, too, has a part to play here. A product of her times, when I tried to tell her what Tom did to me, she, my mother, all powerful, all knowing won't listen and says in complete contradiction of what I know to be so, that he did not. No way sexual abuse exists in families such as ours, that is only for others. For decades I have lived a prey to confusion: if I say x is the case, and someone else says no, it is y, regardless of how clear I have been in my views, I immediately hesitate, unsure, uncertain, maybe I am wrong after all.

Tom, though is more than a merciless judge, he was my first brush with the sexual aspects of the masculine. Months later, with encouragement from Ingrid in another session, I "asked" Tom why he had acted as he did. "You were such a lovely little thing" was his reply. Yes, with my big brown eyes and curly coppery-brown hair that people remarked on, I think I probably was. But wandering on my meditation walks I came to realise that another major psychological consequence of my brush with Tom was my deeply unconscious knowledge that men were dangerously unpredictable and it was not safe to be playfully close. Only then did I finally understand why as a teenager I had been unable to flirt, or relate playfully with boys of my own age. Of no great consequence perhaps; yet I had a fairly empty, almost unhappy adolescence.

In my adult life my friendships with men have been of the good companion, good colleague, Amazon type variety; not a bad thing in the Law Faculty. In shops, though, I would look longingly at frilly blouses, lacy undies and think, "no, not with my sensible face." Tom, it seemed, had sent Aphrodite, with her love of fun, playful flirting, irresponsibility, spontaneity and pampering, into deep hiding. As Ian said when we discussed this "But it was all right, for I found you." Bless him so he did; and many, many happy years of marriage have followed. So it was not a major trauma, far from it; yet I did not have access to all aspects of being a woman.

And as I looked back at that tickling episode, that other brush with the masculine where I had been ridiculed, humiliated and thrown away as useless, I saw a denial of personal power, both physically and emotionally. It was clear to me during that session with Jan, that it was no accident a man was giving me that particular session. I had been wounded, branded by the men in my childhood, albeit completely accidentally in the case of my father. It seemed appropriate that a man should help me make contact with these incidents and help me disentangle myself from the ensuing confusion and distortion.

Turning to Bendigo, my mother's long and inexplicable absence, my brushes with the Ant, I found rejection in many guises. On the one hand, my fear that my mother had rejected, abandoned me; leading, I now understood, to decades of fearing that the people to whom I have offered my affection will suddenly do likewise. And, on the other hand, my own rejection of myself: most obviously that curious, adventure-loving, exploring little imp that is Judith who was so severely criticised for exploring the garden. For years she was visible only in our unconventional holidays: travelling by train across India in a hired railway carriage; Ian and I, free from the restraints of Soviet guides, exploring, again by train, the eastern half of the USSR (as it then was), Mongolia, and Western China. Less obvious, but more important, was the rejection of the totality of myself arising from an obsessive need to be good, to meet the expectations of others; Ant said Mummy wouldn't come back unless I was a good little girl — as she defined it.

Bendigo brought other unsuspected consequences that surfaced in other Rosen sessions: it seemed that only my father remained sure and steady during that time; the one known, trusted protector in a sea of confusion; my rock in times of stress. I saw myself, a toddler of eighteen months, standing in my cot, arms up waiting for Dad to pick me up. Up I go onto his shoulder, nestling in cheek to cheek, ah, now I am safe, now all is well in my little world.

When my father died in 1964 we were living in Phnom Penh, Cambodia. The benefits of grief or bereavement counselling were not widely understood at that time, and certainly not available in Phnom Penh. We went for a week to a cottage on the Gulf of Thailand: to the sea and the seemingly eternal soothing nature of the Cambodian countryside. Thereafter it was life as usual. Only when I did my Rosen training, twenty-five years later, did I realise what his death had meant to me — the almost chronic barely conscious feeling of anxiety, insecurity now that he was no longer available to be my rock in times of stress.[55]

And my birth, what part did my birth and its associated feelings play in my ensuing life? To relive one's birth is a powerful experience; the

---

55 See also *Duck*, p. 105

feelings involved are intense — be they pain, fear, joy, love. In my case the most overwhelming feeling seemed to be fear — fear and more fear. My mother's fear of the pain of childbirth — as it appeared — and later my own fears in the constriction of the vagina.

Ingrid and I speculated that I had taken my mother's fear into my own very new and vulnerable unconscious. Certain it is that to this day I hate dark underground places. My reaction on inspecting an underground mine in Bolivia was almost certainly an unconscious replay of how I had felt in the vagina all those years previously.[56] However, there is more to it than that. For years I have been bedevilled by fear: fear of anything, everything, fear of the unknown, raw fear. I am just frightened, I can't tell you why. It appears that small baby was born into fear and carried it with her for years.

Other consequences of my birth came to me gradually. Pondering the bodywork implications of breast cancer with Jennifer, we speculated that my life-long uncertainty as to when it was appropriate for me to protect my own interests had its origins in that fleeting second's abandonment just after my birth when my mother's needs took priority over mine.

If we go back to the question I asked at the beginning, why did I want to put myself through this spasmodically painful bodywork process? I had certainly stirred memories of childhood incidents that had been painful at the time; in fact, repressed, because the child had found them too painful, too overwhelming to handle. And the recovery of them was also painful. So what could I, did I gain from this process?

Remember that I had no conscious memory of some of these incidents; and of others, I knew the barest outline, and had lost contact with the feelings involved.[57] All I "knew", all that was conscious for me, and even this awareness was diffused at the very edge of my consciousness, was that I had to be "good", was driven to be good in all relationships, in every situation, physically, mentally and morally.

Additionally, it seemed responsibility, leadership, had a tendency to come my way; I was vaguely aware I was considered a "powerful woman". Yet I never felt that power. If I had a position, Sub-Dean of the Law Faculty, wife of the Ambassador, I was all right; I exercised the power that

---

56 This took place in 1978, years before my Rosen training.

57 In a bodywork session two different classes of incidents may surface. In the first, the client has no conscious memory of the situation: the case with the incident with Tom in the sleep-out. In the second, the adult has a memory of the incident, or has been reminded of it, it may be part of the family folklore, but has no memory of the feelings involved. This latter was the case with the death of my baby brother. I knew my mother had been absent for many weeks, but had no memory of any of the feelings involved, rejection, abandonment and so on.

was inherent in the position. But when I was on my own, plain Judith Nicholson, it was as if I did not know the meaning of the word "power". And withal there was this fear, nameless fear, lurking in the wings.

Reviewing all these incidents together I noticed first the outward looking orientation: I was looking always to others to provide support, affirmation, approval, psychological nourishment of one sort or another. It never ever entered my mind I could supply these things for myself. The irony was that at the same time I was telling myself my freedom was important to me. So it seemed I lived a constant paradox. Seeking consciously always to be free and independent, yet unconsciously deeply dependent on others. Confusion must be one of the leitmotivs here, seeing myself through a glass darkly: confusion in the child, confusion in the adult, and confusion between outward appearances and inner feelings. If I gained little else from my Rosen sessions it was clear this insight alone was a pearl beyond price.

Somehow, from somewhere, that woman, Judith, lost touch with feelings of unconditional love. She felt she had to be good in order to be loved, and since she never felt good enough, she never actually felt loved. In my mind, I know this is nonsense, I was a greatly loved and cherished only child at the very heart of my parents' world. I might have known it, but I was some years into my Rosen training before I began to be able to feel that love, and with those recaptured feelings began the first stirrings of love for myself just exactly as I am. Unconditional love for oneself, another veritable pearl of a feeling, making any pain involved in recapturing repressed feelings pale into insignificance.

Would these insights though, be able to help me adjust to the changing circumstances of my life? Looking at the psychological profile I had drawn I was struck by the lack of personal power. Not power in the sense of my capacity to dominate others; but the power that has its roots in feelings of confidence, a value of self, of the legitimate importance of oneself to that self. This is the power that enables, that frees, that is inevitably present in every birth, every change. The woman, Judith, who unconsciously felt she was inadequate, wrong, naughty if she ventured off the beaten track, who had to be good in order to be loved, she who was mysteriously beset by fear, had lost touch with that power which would enable her to seek the freedom to be herself — whatever that self might be. Moreover, she had lost touch with that same power that would enable her to capitalize on that freedom and to do whatever it was that freed self might want to do.

If this conclusion sounds glib, so much "psycho-speak" gleaned from the odd weekend personal growth workshop, remember it has been slowly, patiently and painstakingly pierced together over many years, with much bodywork, some counselling and considerable help and encouragement from supportive family and friends. Only now (in 1998), ten years almost to the day since I set out for Stockholm, an uncertain woman looking for change, has the mirror cleared, the picture become free of distortions. Now I am free to move into clearer sunnier pastures. As Marion Rosen says, bodywork is about possibilities, unknown possibilities, which can bring about change. It did this for me.

PART IV

Hidden Treasure

Then a woman said,
Speak to us of Joy and Sorrow.
And he answered:
Your joy is your sorrow unmasked.
And the selfsame well
From which your laughter rises
Was oftentimes filled with your tears.

Khalil Gibran
The Prophet

Digging for Joy
"What Wouldn't Your Mother Let You Do?"

When I entered Ingrid's room on the third anniversary of my departure from Australia for Sweden, it seemed more beautiful than ever. Physically I was feeling none too bright. I asked her to work my lower abdomen in which there was much tension and some pain. A word floated up as soon as she began, *creativity*.

"What was it," she asked, "your mother wouldn't let you to do?" The answer was instantaneous; "Have ballet lessons". As I spoke, I could see myself as a five-year-old outside my first school jumping, capering about with excitement, "Please, please, may I learn ballet?" "No, I'm sorry you can't." End of story. Those were the post-depression years of the late 1930s; one did not question decisions about spending money. In any event, my Rosen training was establishing that I was a "good girl", and good girls never question their mother's decisions.

I lay on the massage table all those years later watching in stunned surprise the actions of my body. It cramped, convulsed and then went into a deep spasm. Sobs came from a part of me I had never touched before, never even suspected existed, deep, deep within; my constantly frustrated and largely hidden, even from myself, urge to dance.

Ingrid worked quietly on; a theme developed. A book, my unwritten legal book. I had long nurtured a dream that one day I would write a short monograph of simplicity and scholarship on one particular complex legal topic. It was clear now that was never to be. At first with all my family responsibilities there was not sufficient time for the research. Now that I had more time, I realised my topic required a lifetime's experience in that particular area of law. That I did not have and could not now achieve. There was real pain here, a great sense of loss, a nasty feeling of despair. Was my whole life to be spent as the good daughter, the good wife, the good mother, the good colleague, the good citizen? Was there never ever to be time to be just me, to do whatever it was that I wanted to do, freed from the responsibilities of the roles that living my life seemed to have imposed (with my permission)?

I had read in Jung of the *persona*: the mask he says we put on as we play out our roles in dealing with our world — wife, mother, friend, colleague — in most cases, for much of the time, they are just that, roles. We rise in the mornings, put on our costume and act out our play. Some of us identify closely with our roles. We become a driven businessman, a conscientious worker, an almost too loving mother. Others of us are uncertain, the role does not feel right, is not really us, is it supposed to be? Or should we be somewhere else, looking for another role? Even here according to Jung we are identifying with a *persona*, seeing ourselves in terms of a role. The key he says lies in seeing our actions for what they are, a role we may have to, or want to, play; but not all of us. There is, it appears, more to us than our roles.

After my reading of Jung I came to see my diplomatic life as a role, a performance I gave. I put on the appropriate costume — whatever it might be, welcomed my guests, fed, watered, talked to them — asked questions Ian wanted answered. I put as much of myself into that role as felt safe. It was said I had some of the required skills, so I played my part well. People wrote to me, rang me, thanked me for the warm relaxed atmosphere of my hospitality. But for all that it was theatre.

What I had not seen clearly prior to this session was how many other parts of my life were also theatre. I was a good daughter. I did what my loving parents expected of me: good education at tertiary level, a profession so I could develop myself and be independent. I was a good wife. To the best of my ability I tried to be sensible, intelligent, capable and flexible, permitting the growth of a stable family on a global stage. In that role, I was loving and beloved too, that must be said. I was helped, nurtured and protected every step of the way. I identified totally with that role for many years.

I tried to be a good mother, loving, gentle, firm, adamant as required, putting the rearing of my children and their demands ahead of my low profile career as an academic. That career, also, had its demands; the good colleague became Sub-Dean, published legal articles, did all the things good academics do. I took all these roles on: they were offered, I accepted. It was never involuntary.

But at the end of the day, lying on Ingrid's massage table that morning in my mid-fifties, it was clear there was something missing. By almost any standards I had had an excellent life, blessed with so much love, material sufficiency, interest and excitement. But where was the vitality, the joy? Why was it that all I felt was a sort of exhaustion, as if the mere process of living had worn me down and left me drained, dead, disinterested, and possibly boring?

For a few days following this session I was drunk, intoxicated, ecstatic with the heady and rather insubstantial feelings of vitality and creativity that had been stirred. I danced and sparkled my way through a series of mundane chores in the city of Stockholm. Everyone I spoke to smiled at me. I went looking for a postcard for a friend to help me express what I was feeling. I found one, a back view of a beautifully formed tanned bum, glowing with health and life, clad in frothy lace knickers, lilting and tilting off the page! "Yes," I thought, "that's one aspect of how I feel; but no, this friendship will not stand that!" I went to the florist; I would buy a pot plant for my garden room. But no, they were all too straight, too formal. "What do I need?" I asked myself. "Something blazing in the sun, riotous, overflowing, falling, spreading everywhere — a vivid red bougainvillea perhaps, blazing in a tropical garden."

I lived the next few weeks as if on a merry-go-round. Up and down I went: floating, spinning high on feelings of untrammelled creativity; then down, down in the depths of despair that seemed to be surfacing as a result of my session. A despair compounded of feelings of emptiness and a lack of personal fulfilment associated with living my life largely for others. Since Ingrid had left on holiday, I took my seemingly bewitched psyche on long meditation walks. Slowly I realised that I was now experiencing the spiral aspect of the unconscious journey. I had gone up to the heady realms of creativity, and then down in order to see what was standing in my way.[58] Gradually it also became clear that for those magic feelings of creativity and vitality to become permanent, they would have to become personal to me in some way, integrated into particular experiences of my life.

During Ingrid's absence, Karin another skilled Rosen practitioner was giving me one of my twenty-five Rosen sessions, when Tom and his misdoings in my early childhood surfaced again. As she worked, Karin asked a question I had never thought to ask myself, "Did you love him?" Again I watched my body's reaction in stunned surprise. It heaved, convulsed almost, and then I was sobbing uncontrollably, flooded with memories of such happiness, such carefree joy. There I was splashing in the bath, sitting on his lap being read stories, arms around his neck, so safe, so happy, so joyful.

Karin worked quietly on, a connection came up: Tom, who owned an antique shop, used to give me books, old ones with beautiful leather covers, thick creamy coloured paper; not books you read so much as books you handle; the book itself a beautiful piece of craftsmanship. Suddenly I felt joy, my own personal joy, my joy in my books. The books I carry around the world, acquire in bookshops all over the world, have in every room in the house. The books that steady me, comfort me and never let me down.

As Karin moved to work on my legs and feet, I found another of my own joys in life: water, swimming, surfing. O how I hated being in Stockholm, surrounded by the waters of the Baltic, and yet largely unable

---

58 See also *The White Rose*, p. 133 and *The Little Demons*, p. 138 illustrating again the up and down nature of unconscious travel.

to swim. In the winter the water was too cold. I could manage the temperature in the summer, but the fertiliser run-off from the nearby farms sent the water thick with green algae. I tried it once, you couldn't see your feet, it was like swimming in thick slightly salted pea soup. But now as that session progressed I could see myself, feel myself surfing at Point Leo. Ah yes there was joy, another of my own personal joys.

About this time I was invited to be an assistant to my supervisor in two Rosen training workshops. I stood on the first day, moving quietly around the class as the students worked. I made suggestions: hold your hands this way, watch the breath, try this question, try that one. Joy came flooding in, I was teaching, I was teaching! How could I have forgotten the joy that teaching has always brought me?

Later I stood facing the whole class and my supervisor giving a demonstration session of my insights into the basic nature of Rosen Method Bodywork. Again joy flowed in. I had my insight; I was on my feet, teaching again. I looked up and saw interested, expectant, trusting faces. Suddenly I was no longer nervous and lacking in confidence; my skills, my training, my life itself, it seemed, fell into its appointed place. I gave a good session. I gained my supervisor's blessing to take Rosen Method to Australia and work with it alone until help should arrive. That was important for both of us.

What is the theme of this tale? There seem to be three strands involved: creativity, the roles we play, and vitality or joy. Are they but facets of the same jewel? I think so. The core, the jewel must be that spark of creativity, the part of the Divine in all of us, that which makes us unique whatever it may be. Joy and vitality are the feelings which flow from touching that spark. The roles are what we feel constrained to play by our lives and the society in which we live: "the shoulds", "the musts", "the oughts". Joy and vitality are ours, then, as we put aside our roles and touch our own spark, our own essential creative core.

Some months later I was out walking Sabina around an exquisitely beautiful lake when an insight floated up. I need no longer fret about lost creative opportunities — no dancing lessons, an unwritten legal text. They were past, gone. But the future lay ahead. There it seemed I could live my whole life so that it, of itself, would be the most exquisite work of art that I could possibly create. Nothing more, nothing grand, just my own life, my own jewel to cut and polish as I would.

The White Rose

I am feeling confused, a little shaky, and so I seek the clarity, the steadiness that comes to me from the written word. Even as I write, I see a wonderful pair of images — the clarity of the written word and a recent symbol for me, a white rose. It seems that I am now at a central part of my meditative experiences: the relationship of *heart/mind* — *rose/word*.

You will remember that as part of my Rosen training I have to receive sessions given by a professional in front of a small group of fellow students. I had such a session from Lisen, an experienced and wise practitioner and teacher. She was working on my back, in the area of my diaphragm, moving gently, albeit powerfully. In a technical bodywork sense the "connection" was excellent. I felt her touch on my back in every pore of my body.

I started talking slowly and quietly of my recent experiences when staying for a few days in a Benedictine retreat house in the beautiful medieval town of Vadstena, in southern central Sweden. In particular I spoke of the two masses I had attended. One in the former Abbey Church of St Birgitta, now a Lutheran church, and the other in the chapel of the existing Catholic Brigittine Order.

In the Lutheran Church I was flooded with the realisation that I wished no intercessors in my spiritual life. I knew not where this realisation would take me, I knew only that henceforth I would speak to my God, by whatever name, myself in my own language. In the Brigittine chapel watching the heavy crucifix over the sombre altar, the black shrouded nuns praying in attitudes of dutiful submission, I knew suddenly that my spiritual life was one of light, joy and love, not heavy with pain, power and suffering. There were no stained glass windows in the chapel, through a clear window the sun sparkled on the glorious beauty of a Swedish lake in early spring. Here I knew were the images of my spiritual life, the beauty of the Divine world: Sun, Light, and Heart.

Asking me to turn on my back, Lisen started to work my diaphragm again, right at the top under my breasts where the rib cage meets the sternum. She said gently that she felt I had an opening before me that I was resisting by using words to describe what I was feeling. I was quiet for a while. Then, "What will happen to *me* if I go through that opening?" I asked. "Yes," she replied, "it is hard if you lack trust, but you have no need to fear."

I lay quiet a little longer waiting for courage or love to come to carry me through. Then I went; I can't tell you where, but I went through that opening and I found a White Rose, nothing more, just one exquisitely beautiful White Rose. I lay still, gently breathing, holding that White Rose in my vision for a while. Then her hands moved and my mind moved with them. Immediately she said, "You have started to think again, I can feel it with my hands and see it on your face, it has lost that look of deep calm and peace it had before."

So we worked in unison: I would find, hold my Rose and then lose it; she would remind me, I would find it again. Finally she said to me, "There is a power in you that will help you overcome the resistance you set up through using words."

I have had many moving sessions in my Rosen experiences. This would have to be one of the deepest and most beautiful — one that penetrated deep into the core of my being. This is the Ultimate Mystery, if you like. We think we are mind and matter; so we are at one level. But at another level, deep within, it appears I am other, Ineffable, Unknowable, beyond the mind: the Magic of Life, the Mystery of Life. This Other we describe as we can. For me it is Heart, Love, Light, Trust, The Divine, The White Rose — peace and beauty.

The Magic of Life

Dear Friend,

In Sweden I gave two of the Rosen sessions I must give as an intern, in which for both of my clients the central theme was the "Magic" or "Mystery of Life". In one session my client was a member of a Catholic Order now seeking to be released from vows; the other, a young science undergraduate. Each, it seemed, had taken up their particular vocation seeking enlightenment on the magic of life, or the meaning of life as the nun put it. She had expected the Church would assist her in her search. In fact, she said, not only had it not done so, but in the interests of conformity to accepted dogma, it had sought to smother or stifle her own intuitions.

If the Church can't help, maybe science can. Or can it? The young undergraduate was edgy, restless. Science, he was finding, of its very nature names, describes, analyses, proves and thus contains, limits and restricts the possibilities of magic.

Why am I so hung up on all this, just at the moment, Friend? I have known for some time now, that in my quest for meaning in my life, the magic of my life, I do not belong to any known group of believers. I take a piece here, a piece there and experience my own mystery, make sense of my own life, as I live it. There is much freedom here; no one tells me what to experience, what to believe, except me. There is no one to correct me or support me; I have to stand alone taking responsibility for my own views. Freedom as always is double-edged.

From the Yogis I have accepted that eventually I will go, as they put it, beyond the mind. I can experience this state now; it is very beautiful, wondrous in fact. The world is full of possibilities; life becomes rich, varied, full of tone and texture. To go beyond the mind in this way is to travel to that place where Judith melts into the Magic, her version of the Magic, her Divine. Here, she both is, and, is not. The ultimate paradox:

she has to be, in order to know that she is not.

Heavens, Friend, I doubt you have followed me this far. I know what I mean; I know what I have experienced. Will I ever be able to put it into words? Should I even be trying? Am I, too, about to try to define, analyse, describe and so limit and restrict my own Magic, my own Divine? Maybe I just have to remember that what I write of my Divine is the point from which I jump off, not a boundary fence which encloses me.

Is it as simple as that? I wonder…?

The Little Demons

Dear Friend,

I recall my meeting with my exquisite White Rose, who could forget her? Well a few weeks later I had an "encounter" with another fragment of my unconscious, one which I can only describe as the "Little Demons".[59] Ian was away for a week at a conference in Paris; I was alone in our big house on the out-skirts of Stockholm. I awoke with a start in the middle of the night to the gripping image of a group of small, evil looking men in black-hooded cloaks, bearing two-pronged forks, about to climb into bed with me! I know this sounds like the fantasies of some psychotic; but it happened to me, and I feel quite sane.

Quickly, sharply, I pulled myself together and told them to hop it one and all. I had met the White Rose, I said, and therefore had no room for them in my life. Since Ian, the steadying rock in my life was not around; I went down to the kitchen for the inevitable cup of tea.

In the morning I rang dear, imperturbable Amy. "What a coincidence," she said, "I have just been reading about similar encounters in a Tantra on Yoga!" The import of the remainder of our talk was that this imagery must have been symbolising my own personal demons and that in due course I would have to deal with these — accept them and integrate them into my psyche at every level. For, she said, in Yoga terms, the good and the bad are all part of the One. Similarly I knew from my reading in psychology that one has to meet the contents of one's "shadow" and, gradually accepting them, integrate them into one's psyche.

Perhaps I should add that on this first encounter I did not relate the imagery to myself personally in any way. In all honesty I think I was so shocked I didn't even try. Had you asked me previously, I would have said that I did not believe in the concept of the Devil, a concept I had thought of in terms of unrelieved, unmitigated evil. Yet my unconscious

---

[59] See *The Witchdoctor*, p. 22 and *Digging for Joy*, p. 127 for a description of the up and down, spiral, nature of unconscious travel.

for its own good reasons, no doubt, had selected symbols universally recognised as associated with the devil — black-hooded people bearing two-pronged forks.[60]

I was shaky that next day, very shaky; it was clear that yet again something in my unconscious had been deeply moved. Since it was a day of Rosen training, I stayed near my closest Rosen mate all day; then slept the next night in the warmth and earthy comfort of the house of a close Canadian friend.

We now move forward about three weeks. Night again, I awake with an acute pain between my shoulder blades. As I ease them there is a zrrrp of movement and suddenly I am confronting an image of my own personal judge in my unconscious. Looking into his face, listening to what he is saying, suddenly I understand that with his twisting distortion of my view of myself he is a demon figure, my own personal version of the devil, perhaps. Despite my stunned surprise, I try to do as Amy has suggested — stay firm and attempt a conversation.

"OK," I say, "I accept that a judge, an entity who helps me discriminate and differentiate is a necessary part of my psyche; but surely you don't have to be such an unmitigatedly negative judge. All you have ever done is carp, criticise and condemn. You say I am not good enough, I can't cope; I am second rate, inadequate. This undermines me, subverts me: makes it impossible for me to lead the life I now know is available."

"Why don't you help me accept the gifts my spiritual life seems to be offering: to be able to live love in some way I don't yet fully understand. To live love, as I now see it, I must be able both to give and receive it. With your constant insidious carping and criticism you make this well nigh impossible. I listen to you, I never think to doubt you, and so I reject myself and fear the rejection of others. Thus bewitched, I can neither offer love freely, nor accept it readily."

There was more in this vein which I cannot now recall. I do remember arguing passionately at one stage, "Love is my birthright, you cannot deny me that."

As I write it seems a fantastic experience, empty of impact; nothing

---

60 See, *The Witchdoctor*, p. 22 for a description of the use of symbolic language by the unconscious

could be further from the truth. It was a conversation of passionate intensity, in, for me, a scene of total reality. With every fibre of my being I was pleading, pleading with my demon detractor, that he now pull with me and help me go forward in peace to fulfil my destiny. The morning brought such silence, such an *absence of tension*, such peace, such portents of joy.

Perhaps I had won.

Beloved...Ah, Beloved — Reflection

I have hesitated to write this last month. This silence bothers me, for it comes not from an absence of anything to say, but rather from a hesitancy to put pen to paper for fear of being misunderstood.

What is it that could be so easily misunderstood? Why the word *love*, of course, one of the most used and abused words in the English language, meaning something different for every person who uses it, and carrying a different meaning for the same person on differing occasions, like as not. A veritable minefield of a word. It is curious isn't it, that for all the multitude of feelings involved, the English language should have only one word.

The Jungian writers distinguish carefully between two states, *being* or *falling in love* with someone, and loving someone. In their view, the first is often a forerunner of the second. Mary falls in love with John, later she may come to love him. In Jungian terms the first involves Mary's projections onto John and may therefore be unreal, not linked to John as the person he is in reality. Mary is in love with John "because he is so gentle and caring," that is she has projected on to him what she is unconsciously seeking in a male partner. The duration of this relationship will depend on the extent to which John's actual personality matches

Mary's projections. If they do, all may be well; if not, then it is founded on sand, unreality and Mary (and John) are most likely fated for unhappiness.

In Jungian terms, however, if Mary loves John, then she is loving him as he is. She is operating in a real, or relatively real world. Both she and John have a fair chance of happiness if their love is mutual and if their expectations of love are, at least, compatible. The word expectations seems important here. I went wandering in the forest musing on all this. The word that came to mind was contract, with some terms explicit and many implicit. Couples in this day who marry, or who agree to live together, agree on the general outlines of their relationship. Even if it is the generalised "love, honour and obey" the agreement is there, and it is mutual. This is, and should, be reciprocal love. Two people agree to love each other, to live together, to beget or not beget children together. They agree in effect to a lifetime of joint ventures, thus doing many things together neither can do alone. You love me, and I love you. You stop loving me and I will probably stop loving you because I am hurt, rejected, angry, frustrated and jealous.

Now where does *beloved* fit into this and why do I find it such an incredibly powerful word? I suppose because it brings me to feelings of Divine Love. Curious that there should be no widely known word in English to describe these feelings. The phrase "brotherly love" is used. I find it, unsatisfactory, not because it is sexist — I would find sisterly equally so — but because to me it seems vapid, empty of content. The mystical texts use the word "agape" derived from a Greek word meaning brotherly love. I can't relate to that word at all, and yet, over the years of my meditation and bodywork, I have been delving more and more deeply into the mysteries of Divine Love.

However, if instead of writing beloved, I write *be-loved* then I am describing a feeling that is becoming known to me and which I describe as Divine Love. There are two aspects of this: first, the feelings, which I have towards any person, I hold be-loved; and secondly the feelings I have myself when I feel that I am be-loved. In each case the operative part of the word is "be", being loved, nothing more. There is no contract here, no expectations, nothing mutual; nothing, in fact, that says that two people have to be involved.

If John is be-loved of Mary, then all John has to do is "be", to exist; by his very being, in his very being, he is loved. His existence, nothing more, enriches Mary's life in countless ways of which he may not even be aware.

I used the word be-loved not so long ago. I used it, casually almost, to another and I used it with this meaning. As I did so I felt the freedom involved, unconditional love, freedom in love, a very tall order. The word came and went, feelings came and went with it, but nothing, not one thing was required of anybody — just to be, to be loved, to be *be-loved.*

Later, as is often the way, I lay quietly in bed that night and felt what it was like to be be-loved of another, or possibly even of myself. Here was magic, the freedom, the peace. I could be absolutely still; not strive nor strain; not feel I must, I must not; I should, should not; why didn't I, why can't I. Nothing. I just am, the feeling says, exactly as I am, every minute of every day with a constantly changing kaleidoscope of actions and feelings. And, just exactly as I am, so I am be-loved. This is a beautiful feeling. Curious that, I won't seek the reasons; I will just leave it at that.

The Dancer Within

Dear Friend,

Hello, I am just back from three days cruising on a Russian ship from Helsinki to Leningrad (now St Petersburg) and back. Initially I was unenthusiastic about this trip, feeling that my days of conducted tours of museums and palaces with crowds of other tourists were well and truly over. However, Ian was keen, he had long wanted to see the famous collection of Impressionist paintings at The Hermitage and this seemed like a good opportunity. As we talked, I suddenly discovered a previously unknown desire to visit the Kirov Theatre. Decision made, it was marvellous how everything fell into place. A Swedish friend living there was able to buy us the theatre tickets. Our Russian tour leader did not demure when we asked permission to leave the group for the evening. Although this did give us a long walk alone across a foreign city to find the theatre, and a twelve and a half hour day away from the boat with only a few drinks and one rather scanty Russian meal.

How I loved that theatre, no sooner had I walked in the door than something about it grabbed me. Although it is similar in concept and decor to Covent Garden in London, it is lighter, more elegant, more gracious in a way, with a beautiful deep mid-blue colour scheme embellished with gold and silver; rich, light and peaceful at the same time. I can see the deep folds of the heavy silk brocade curtains, feel and sense the atmosphere even now as I write.

I had hoped to see ballet, but the evening's performance was the opera *Boris Godunov*, beautifully sung, staged, produced and dressed. We left at interval, though, overborne with doom and gloom, fatigue and hunger. So back to the boat, an overnight trip to Helsinki and a return flight to Stockholm.

Although I had been clearly moved in some way by the theatre, I was nevertheless stunned to spend the rest of that night on board sleepless, living and reliving my apparently never-ending capacity to fear rejection by those to whom I have offered my affection. I lay watching myself, I saw this demon that lurks in so many of my thoughts, actions and reactions. I could scarcely credit my own feelings: how could I be so crazy, allow myself to be so manipulated (for it is manipulation by unconscious forces we must be talking of here)? How could a woman who has lived a life so rich in love be so powerless in the face of these feelings? I felt so incredibly vulnerable I wished I could die.

Back in Stockholm a long day loomed. Ian went back to the office and I could see myself alone all day in the house, tired and achy from a lack of sleep and a prey to these tearing feelings. I thought, I just can't face that, anything but that, so to steady myself I popped Sabina into the car and set off for what I call my circuit walk. Although less pretty than some of my walks, I usually find its beautiful old birch and pine trees calming and steadying. Two things I really needed that day.

Walking slowly, I started a conversation in my head about the Kirov Theatre: there seemed to be something about the curtain with its so-beautifully-embroidered rich heavy brocade folds. What did it have to do with me and my unconscious? Was it the colour, that deep rich blue is one of my favourite colours? Was it the richness of the embroidery; I am a very tactile person, texture in embroidery always attracts me; or was the curtain itself symbolic of something? What was my unconscious trying to tell me?

Suddenly I was no longer musing on the curtain. There shimmering on the path in front of me, as if from nowhere, was a dancer, a prima ballerina, a woman of great beauty and brilliance, dancing exquisitely before my very eyes on a deserted path in a Swedish wood. I fell silent, stopped walking and, shaking slightly, sat on a nearby rock. I was tremulous and full of wonder. It seemed I *knew* that dancer, knew all about her, her thoughts, her feelings, her very being; she was within, deep within me somewhere. I felt as if I was that dancer, she was me, we were as one. Come dance with me…

As I sat quietly watching, an intuition floated up: this was a dancer beloved by her audiences less for her technical skills than for her wondrous ability to portray feelings through dance, and to evoke those same feelings in others. I asked a question: Why did she dance? Was it money, status, stardom, a sense of duty, a "should" or an "ought"? The answer was swift and sure: dancing was her life, she loved to dance, was passionate about dancing, danced for the sheer joy of living. Ah, she was free then, free in her dancing.

What can I say, Friend? It was an experience beyond words. As I write, I am filled with a wondrous joy at the beauty and the powerful simplicity of that encounter.

My dancer within...

The Little Mermaid — A Gorgeous Holiday

Dear Friend,

Just at the moment, my life seems to be flooding in, out, in, out, quite out of control, a wondrous feeling, a little shake-making nonetheless.

Why am I shaky today, tremulous, in fact? *Freedom*, in a word, sister to *Joy*, and one of the most wonderfully, gloriously, marvellous feelings I have come across. I am drunk with it, intoxicated with it, bursting with it. I want to sing, dance, run naked in the streets whooping and yelling. I can't actually think how to express it at the moment. I wish I could; everything I consider seems inadequate somehow. Words like rollicking come to mind. I don't seem able to rollick, what a hoot!

It is about a month now since a glorious young mermaid erupted out of my unconscious onto the massage table. She was the most exquisite creature you ever saw. Hair of spun gold, glimmering in the sun; lithe, elegant, blue/green body, dancing, gambolling, playing with the ocean, in, out, up, down, over and under. The beauty of the scene, the frolics, the joy, the freedom, ah the freedom... "Be-loved by all, beholden to none," I whispered to Ingrid as I watched.

Later during two sparkling weeks in London I began to live that freedom. Oh, the feelings, those exquisite feelings as I came and went, free at every level. I was staying with a close friend in a wonderfully convenient flat in Chelsea. This combination meant I was lovingly supported, well situated, yet could come and go as I chose. I didn't shop, not much, nor "do the shows". I simply floated, drifted around London, by every available means of public transport, seeing old friends and making new ones.

Freedom surfaced at every point. I saw Foreign Affairs friends of long standing, listened to the well-known chatter and felt free. This would soon no longer be my world; I could just let it go. It had been very good to me, I had enjoyed much of it; but it was time to move on.

I gave Rosen Bodywork sessions and talked much of Rosen work to people who came my way. I am beginning to see this as a recurring pattern in my life. The teacher again, perhaps; not expounding at a lectern this time, simply living my life and talking of what I have experienced.

Then I spent time walking, talking, driving, and dining with a new friend. There were new feelings here, beautiful feelings; feelings I realise I have never experienced before. Feelings of freedom in friendship, freedom in offering and receiving affection. As I look back down my life there have been my feelings of inadequacy, my fears of rejection, my inability to trust and my need to be dependent. All of these, largely unconscious, have made feelings of freedom in friendship well nigh impossible. And now, a priceless gift. The offer of a friendship that is not a whit less precious, but which, for some reason, is not bedevilled by the customary nasties. What joy! What a simply lovely holiday, a taste of things to come, perhaps...

Since my return to Stockholm, Sabina and I have resumed our summer wanderings- her gambols and my reflections. Looking back I now realise I have been absolutely addicted to, drugged by, in bondage to — whatever word you want to use — the need to be loved and to be able to love in turn. In this I was like any other addict, totally dependent on my fix — love, approval — I just craved it, had to have it. This was programmed into my being, so programmed that it was unthinkable for me to live any other way; and equally unthinkable for me that others would be able, or want, to live differently.

The other aspect I now see, was, and this has a devilish quirk, that although I constantly craved love, it was difficult for me to detect it when it was present. This will sound daft to you, I know. It does to me. Yet, as I have lived and re-experienced aspects of my life these last few years, I promise you it is true. It was my fate, my karma as the Yogis would say, to live a life rich in love, abundant in love, and yet never to be able to "hear" it, to "feel" it until quite recently.

You must be getting restive now. I said I was writing about freedom, instead I appear to be writing of bondage. I am also writing what might appear rubbish. Yet, I assure you, I have never felt more sane, more intelligent, and more on top of my life than I do at the moment. And of even greater surprise, I have never felt less hassled, more free. For with the awareness or understanding of this bondage, has come a realisation of the inner workings of myself — what it is that has driven me to think, feel and operate as I do.

In the Yoga books I have been reading these last few years, the terms realisation and self-realisation carry a subtlety of meaning beyond my grasp. Yet wandering through the forests these last few weeks, a lovely congruence of meaning around the word *realisation* drifted into my mind. Having bodywork sessions, delving deeply into my unconscious, unearthing my past and more general symbolic imagery, I have *realised*, in the sense of, *become aware of*, the restrictions of those old patterns. In so doing, it seems it would now be possible for me to *realise* myself, that is make real the core of my personality. And finally, this in turn now sets up the possibility of *self-realisation*, in the sense of being able to make capital out of the assets of myself, being able to use my own gifts, whatever they may be, freely, joyously, peacefully.

Heavens, perhaps that is what each of us is supposed to do as our appointed task in life, realise our selves and our bondage, and then "realise" our potential.

Can it really be as simple as that?

PART V

Reflections

"Is my contact with others
anything more than a contact with reflections?
Who or what can give me the power
to transform the mirror into a doorway?"

Dag Hammarskjold
Markings

The Mirror of Life

M*arion Rosen and all my Rosen teachers had talked much of reflection:* reflection was the key used to make contact with the unconscious by means of the body. I was to use my hands to reflect to my client the tension or holding in her body, to use words to reflect to her what she had said. Then during my sessions with Ingrid she introduced reflection in another context that would enable me to use the living of my everyday life to maintain contact with my unconscious. Although this was not formally part of my Rosen training it became highly relevant when I returned to Australia as the only Rosen practitioner in the country.

"Look at those incidents in your everyday life, no matter how apparently trivial," Ingrid said, "which you don't seem able to forget, which haunt you as you try to go to sleep, pulling at you in some way. They are hooking onto something in your unconscious, reflecting something, linking your everyday life and your unconscious in some way." Thus she introduced me to what I have come to call the mirror of life…

I had gone to see her that day in 1991 "hooked" on a trivial accident I had had in my car the preceding evening, hooked in particular by feelings of inadequacy and foolishness. Driving home at dusk I had missed my way. Turning to retrace my steps, the rear wheels of my car went off the road; suddenly, unexpectedly, I was balanced precariously over a deep water-filled ditch. What had been a pleasant lazy chat over coffee with a friend, became a quiet drama as I sought help from a neighbouring house, alerted Ian to my plight and asked his office to ring the Swedish Automobile Association — all the time feeling like a complete fool. Who does a U-turn on a quiet suburban road and ends up suspended over a ditch of water for heaven's sake?

And so Ingrid introduced me to the mirror: whom had I been visiting, she wanted to know; what aspect of myself would my friend have been reflecting to me, and, most importantly, what symbolism could I see for myself in my actions and reactions around what had happened to my car?

I wriggled and squirmed as she probed, for my answers revealed that although perfectly capable of extricating myself from that situation, I had opted to have Ian and his office organise the help for me. I could have rung the Automobile Association myself and probably been back home none the worse for wear before Ian even returned from work. At the time I told myself that the telephonist at the AA might not speak enough English; but in my heart of hearts I knew this was unlikely. So what was the mirror showing me, Ingrid wanted to know? That I often chose not to exercise my own power preferring to ask others to exercise theirs on my behalf, was the reply I knew I had to make. Was this a sin? No, not at all, but the inescapable conclusion was that I was unnecessarily burdening others and unnecessarily restraining my own freedom. No wonder I felt foolish.

Handling the mirror of life takes time and practice. At first I saw only the most obvious superficial reflections, that of a one to one archetypal situation. I could recognise an uncomfortable discussion with a teacher for example (an authority figure), as a situation in which a record of my confusion at mother's response to Tom's misdoings was replaying, so that even now it is very easy for me to feel that my views are wrong.

Then with Ingrid's help I begin to look further, to see everyday apparently trivial incidents as reflections also. I was deep in the psychological processes of my Rosen training at that time; "stuff" was surfacing from my unconscious at a great rate. We looked at that car incident again. Was the car suspended over a water-filled ditch showing me that I too was suspended over the ditch of my unconscious — water being a powerful symbol for the unconscious? If so, I would have to practise exercising my own power to pull myself out. For I alone could extricate me from the entanglements of my own unconscious stuff.

The most important reflection of all, though, is that of a persistently recurring image which is almost certainly reflecting something I have unconsciously learnt to do to myself. If I was always seeing others condemning and rejecting me then, suggested Ingrid, I needed to ask myself was I, in some part of my life, unconsciously condemning and rejecting myself?

At this point, the focus shifts: the childhood incidents and the hooking trivia become important in that they show what I am now doing to myself. I am the one rejecting, condemning, and I am rejecting and condemning me, thus denying myself my own power. There need be no projections on others, no resort to victimisation, no denial of power. This is my problem, my responsibility and again I have to handle it myself.[61]

In many ways it is only now, writing of the mirror with the hindsight acquired by many years practice, that I have come to understand all the implications of trying to live this way. It is the reflections in the mirror that have coaxed me to apply all that I learned of myself in my Rosen work to the living of my life, gaining continual practice in recognising old patterns of behaviour, and exercising choices around possible new ones.

I once heard Marion Rosen say she thought there were four stages in the release of old childhood patterns. First in a Rosen session, you see the situation which gave rise to the feeling — incident and associated feelings move from the unconscious to the conscious mind. You are now aware that, for you, this is an emotionally charged and delicate area. Secondly, you recognise after the event, that you acted out the old pattern again. "Zzzt," you say to yourself, "there I go again, alway confused around authority, acting out that old pattern." "This is progress, don't forget," Marion said, "for at least you saw the repeating pattern, only you were too

[61] In fact, what others are allegedly doing to us and what we are doing to ourselves are reflected simultaneously in the mirror. However, often we only see the self-reflection at a later date when we have stopped fretting about what others are doing to us.

late to avoid it." Thirdly, you see the pattern as you are in the midst of it. "Whoops," you say to yourself, "here I go assuming that I must be wrong"; but this time, with luck you can change course and exercise another choice mid-stream. Fourthly, you recognise a situation as being a danger zone for you before it arises. "Watch it," you say to yourself, "I could easily react in that same old way, but with care I can try something different." And finally, a fifth stage if you like — the situation does not arise! Quietly, quietly, patience with the mirror of life...

To be able to change old patterns of behaviour it appeared I needed to apply what I had learnt and then to practise, practise, practise. I am reminded of a student I once saw when I was Sub-Dean of the Law Faculty. He had just failed all his exams and came storming into my room, a bundle of loose-leaf folders under his arm. "Look," he said, "look at all these summaries I made of the lectures and suggested reading. I know all the law, how can I have failed?" I looked at his examination results and the comments of his examiners. "It's possible you know the theory of the law," I replied, "but the examiners all state that you have not applied that knowledge to the facts of the problems you were asked to solve. Not only do lawyers have to know the law, but just as importantly they have to be able to apply that knowledge to the resolution of particular problems."

As in the law, so in my life apparently, application of knowledge was of prime importance. I had to learn to apply what I had learnt, otherwise that knowledge was of no real use to me. The mirror of life...

Jung, too, writes of application and practice. He realised, he says, when he first met the contents of his unconscious, that in seeking deeper contact with it, he needed to personify his feelings in some way, bring them into relationship with his conscious mind and realise them in his life.[62] He used the term synchronicity for that quirk of fate which ensures the circumstances of an old unwanted pattern keep repeating in the mirror of our lives, pointing the way to new learning, other choices.[63]

The most obvious aspect of the mirror is often overlooked, the need to be absolutely still — self-acceptance or in psychological terms a recognition and acceptance of the shadow. If I pull against myself twisting

---

62 C.G. Jung, *Memories, Dreams and Reflections*, Flamingo, London, 1985, pp. 213-218

63 Jung refers to this phenomenon, in which things manifest by laws of correspondence rather than the laws of cause and effect as synchronicity. See Edward C. Whitmont, *The Symbolic Quest*, Princeton University Press, Princeton, 1978.

this way and that, then the mirror can reflect only darkness, confusion and distortion. Could I be kind and gentle to myself, Ingrid asked? Could I try to remember that no one knew what it was like to be me, except me? That would be a first step in no longer whipping myself for feelings of which I was ashamed, the first step in being still, in self acceptance. Ultimately, it seems, change can only occur when I am able to be still within myself. For so long as I fight myself, run from myself, I can't see accurate helpful reflections and there is no foundation, no steady ground beneath me, from which to move. So ironically it is acceptance which lays the ground for change. Put that way it is incredibly simple, almost axiomatic, and yet it makes great sense.

Slowly, as weeks turned to months, to years, I found those former limiting feelings losing some of their power, although the most deeply rooted have remained always as tender spots, danger zones. Constant practice has brought stirrings of new feelings offering possibilities of a new way of living; has proved, for example, that even confrontation, one of my greatest terrors, need not always bring the expected disaster, but can provide some much needed clearing of the air. When the body-psyche stands as still as it dares and correctly interprets the intensity of the hooking incident, it brings about its own changes, its own transformation.

If I accept the existence of the mirror, then logically, conceptually, I must accept that it reflects all life, all of the unconscious, not simply limiting situations from childhood, but including negative self-perceptions. Some years after our arrival in Tumut, wandering through our beautiful rose garden one early spring morning, I looked at the strong healthy plants, glossy leaves, tall straight stems, vibrant gleaming blooms. This had been our project, Ian's and mine, this beautiful spiral-shaped formal rose-garden, with its ninety-nine roses all blending together harmoniously. The form was suggested by Bridget, our landscape architect youngest daughter, and the blending of the colours of the bushes by Leith, a close artist friend.

The whole garden project was one on which family and close friends had worked together for over eighteen months pooling all our different skills. Physically not all that strong at the time, I had offered my enabling, researching, coordinating strengths, collecting together all the required materials, thus allowing the paths, pool and fountain, stands for the climbers and our centre-piece — the beautiful flowing rose *Awakening* — to be constructed by others. For many, many hours that rose-garden had its hooks into me. Was it, I now wonder, telling me something of my psyche, also something of the different psyches of all participants perhaps, if they stopped to glimpse the reflections. It was a lovely thought...

The second half of my book tells the story of my life near Tumut following our return to Australia in late 1991. As I lived my new life, helping Ian develop the farm, planning the garden, building the yurt (the retreat cottage), my Rosen practice and finally the Rosen practitioner training program, in the absence of Rosen sessions, I began to use pain, disease in different parts of my body and the mirror in earnest to help me disentangle myself from all the entangling unconscious material.[64] Initially I used the mirror alone which is never an easy process; later I was blessed to find Jennifer a wise and fun-loving Canberra-based counsellor who herself used the mirror. Then we were able to hold it for each other and help one another carefully identify the reflections.

At first I imagined that the source of the power to turn that mirror into a doorway (be it my body or the circumstances of my life) must be my deeply abiding desire to become free. Later events were to show that the seeds of freedom themselves lay shrouded in the folds of acceptance — acceptance of myself and acceptance of those "nasties" the Universe saw fit to deal me.[65] The mirror of life...

---

[64] See *Snakes in the Grass*, p. 76

[65] See *The Cancer Saga*, p. 201

A Broader Canvas

When *in December 1991 Ian and I returned to Australia,* we were stepping away from the known patterns of Foreign Affairs life after thirty-six years into a complete change of lifestyle. It was another "leap in the dark".[66] An important part of this change for me was the abrupt and total loss of contact with my Rosen world. I had completed my training in Stockholm, was a certified Rosen Method Bodywork practitioner with my certificate from the Rosen Institute in California in my luggage. I was, however, the only Rosen practitioner on the Australian continent with no possibility of further Rosen sessions in the foreseeable future.

I found it unthinkable that I should lose contact with my unconscious world, with the wisdom, the insights, the joy, the richness and the variety of texture and tone it had brought into my life. Life with my unconscious was like a subtly hued three-dimensional film; in contrast life without it was an old drab black and white movie. Trained as I now was in bodywork, traditional verbal therapy had little appeal. Yet I had no knowledge of the general bodywork scene in Australia, and in any event, it was not easy to access from Tumut.

In those circumstances I started to read more and more widely of the general bodywork scene in the United States of America, and

[66] See, Part VI, *Tumut: Building a Dream*, p. 165

simultaneously began to pay even more particular attention to my own body in every aspect of my everyday life, to try to hear what it might be trying to tell me. I remembered *Healing and Wholeness*[67], which Amy had first lent me in 1986 with Sanford's view that pain could have a role in all our lives: that in sending pain, the unconscious, through the body, is trying to catch our attention, to send a message — to protect us, to warn us in some way.

Perhaps, I thought, since I could no longer have regular Rosen sessions, I could at least use the pain or discomfort in my body to help me contact my unconscious. And so very gradually I sought to understand the role of the pain in my life at any particular time. Now many years later, I have come to regard pain as a signpost, a marker along my way as I travel an uncertain route to a hazy destination — a pathfinder. I could also describe it as a roadblock at a junction. There I stay attempting every route until the pain lifts: "Ah that must be my road," I say to myself. Talking to pain, listening to my body...

The fact that once in Tumut I put a greater emphasis for myself on pain than on muscle tension, in no way detracted from my acceptance of Marion Rosen's basic teaching. Although our teachers had talked in general terms of muscle tension as an indicator of holding in the body and blockages, pain is often, although not necessarily, present in these circumstances. Muscle tension is merely one indicator of holding in the body, pain is another.

As I started to pay greater attention to my body in those early Tumut days, I realised that it was talking to me all the time, quietly making suggestions about all aspects of my life. Slowly I learnt to listen and to value its subtle accuracy, its sensitivity and its wisdom. In 1992 just after our move to Tumut, I went to see a recommended GP for a tetanus injection. I was a new patient, he was thorough: he took me through my medical history, how Ian's retirement and the move to Tumut were affecting me, my fairly constant feeling of fatigue. He asked if I would consider Hormone Replacement Therapy: it could help with fatigue, he said, there were no contra-indications in my medical history. I appreciated

---

67 John A. Sanford, *Healing and Wholeness*, Paulist Press, New York, 1977

his care, listened openly to his logical, commonsense arguments; but no, I thought not.

I saw his partner in early 1993 and HRT surfaced again. I was lent a video, given a prescription for low-dose patches; Ian was murmuring in favour, "If it will help with feeling so tired, why not give it a go?" I bought the patches, looked at them, my body, my intuition, shouting insistently "no, no, no." I put them in the drawer of my bedside table and left them there. Some months later routine tests disclosed a small malignant breast tumour. "How lucky your never touched that HRT", murmured the specialist, "goodness only knows what effect that additional oestrogen would have had on your tumour."

When in 1993 cancer came my way, breast cancer at first and then in 1996, acute myeloid leukaemia (cancer of the bone marrow), I turned again to Sanford's talk of disease, as a lack of ease in particular areas of the body and, asking myself the function of breasts or bone marrow in the body, tried to relate that lack of ease in a physical function to my psychological profile as I understood it.[68] This was in effect to treat cancer as another form of bodywork.

In so doing, although I moved beyond the strict teaching of my bodywork training, I simply took the principles I had learnt and applied them on a broader canvas. When we studied "experiential", or "Rosen" anatomy, we were trained to take the physical function of a particular muscle and look for a related emotional content. So, for instance, the rhomboid muscles, those which lie between the shoulder blades close to the surface on the back, one of whose physical functions is to allow the arms to bring something towards you, have a related emotional content — hugging.

Now on my broader canvas, I looked to the function of breasts and bone marrow. None of this is new, although much of it is unknown to conventional Western medicine. Chinese medicine has long connected particular feelings with particular organs of the body. Indian, Ayurvedic, medicine has a large body of knowledge around personality types and tendency to illness. Modern bodywork modalities in the United States of

---

[68] See, Part VII *A Cancer Saga*, p. 201 and Part VIII *Dancing with Death*, p. 251

America and Europe are working each in their own way establishing relationships between a lack of ease, or pain in the body and the unconscious.[69] Many osteopaths, chiropractors and naturopaths build general principles of this knowledge into their work. Many regard the body-mind not as a connection but as a continuum — the important thing is the blockage, sometimes you see it in the body, sometimes in the mind, but it is the same blockage.

And so in the 1990s, wishing to maintain my contact with my unconscious without the assistance of regular Rosen sessions, searching to handle the cancer that erupted in my life consistently with my bodywork philosophy, I moved to this broader canvas. Almost imperceptibly, I began to treat pain and the functions of particular areas of the body as places of possible reflections or metaphors from my body warning of hitherto unrecognised areas of lack of harmony in my unconscious.

69 See bibliography for a short list of relevant books.

PART VI

Tumut
Building a Dream

"I feel a great need for a house
And, even more importantly, a garden of my own;
One that is mine to nurture for eternity.
And I just know I have to grow roses.
My mother's death was all about roses for me.
White roses for the eternally living spirit within all of us;
Red roses for the power, the strength and the courage to live."[70]

Judith Nicholson

[70] In a letter written a few months after my mother's death to a close friend with a passion for gardens.

Turning Points

O*ne Sunday afternoon in Stockholm in late October 1989* our two younger daughters rang. Gan-Gan, my mother, had gone into hospital for "tests", they said, and although there did not seem to be anything specific the matter, she did not seem well and the doctor was concerned. So it appeared was the finely tuned intuition of Bridget, our youngest daughter. "I'm worried, Mum," she said, "I just feel she may never leave hospital, that she may die. Can you come, it feels like a lot for us to handle?" Three days and many phone calls later I was on a plane returning to Melbourne. Thirty-six hours later my mother died quietly and unexpectedly.

Heart failure was the stated cause of death. Those of us who loved her knew that whatever the state of her physical heart, her emotional heart had suffered a mortal blow eighteen months earlier when a combination of failing memory and physical strength had forced the decision that she leave her beloved "Binowee" at Flinders.[71]

Although her room in the hostel in Melbourne was spacious, warm and sunny, bright with all her most treasured possessions, although family and friends visited, took her out, phoned and wrote, we knew she hated it. Hated being so hemmed in, regimented and powerless with the accompanying loss of dignity. She battled gamely to re-establish herself for

---

71 My parent's house at Flinders which was sold in 1988 was the original "Binowee". Later Ian and I named our Tumut property "Binowee". Both houses overlooked water, the aboriginal meaning of the word according to my father; both offered a beautiful place in which to recuperate from the demands of living.

a few months, but in the end found she had neither the strength nor the requisite will to live.

When I arrived in Melbourne she was no longer able to speak. So I sat by her bed for those last thirty-six hours, thinking quietly to myself those things that I would like to have said. First and foremost would have to be “thank you”. Thank you for my life, for a chance to live with you, love you, share your sense of adventure, your sense of fun. I paused then and wondered, how would I, could I ever survive without her. True my Rosen training had unearthed times when she was not as present as the child in me would have wished. But in my adult life she had stood firmly behind me, unstintingly offering loving, wise support as I struggled to raise four young children without any of the help that is available now. As I sat there, I could see the two of us years earlier, my father had died, Ian was away. “Don’t worry, Babe,” she was saying, “our men may sometimes be away when we need them, but we will survive, we are a tough old pair!”

And now as I sit in the hospital one of that tough old pair needs to move on. I feel a moment of panic: life without “Mum”. Yet she is old, tired, and too frail now to live the active, participating life she used to love so much. I know that. I know I can’t ask her to continue to live any longer just for me. It is my turn now to offer her the freedom to die, if that is what she wants, in the same way she had offered me the freedom to live my own life as an adult. And so quietly, gently, we said goodbye and a few hours later she died peacefully in her sleep.

On return to Stockholm I was ill: my eyes clogged with conjunctivitis on waking, almost no voice and a nasty bout of bronchitis. For a few days I lay huddled in my bed ill, exhausted and confused. There followed a really nasty patch. Suddenly I felt so alone in the world: no parents, no siblings, no one with whom I could recall my childhood. It was as if a great chunk of my life died with my mother.

Even worse were my feelings that she had abandoned me: that I was now adrift in the world, belonging nowhere. This sounds illogical, nonsensical almost. Ian and I owned a family house in Canberra that we had bought as the one place we could all call home in all our wanderings. Yet it now appeared, that during all my travels with Ian, irrespective of where we may have been living physically or the existence of our own house in Canberra, unconsciously I had been firmly rooted wherever my mother was living, first at Flinders, and more recently in her lovely room at the hostel. Suddenly I felt I could no longer handle the constant upheavals of our diplomatic life. I wanted to find my place, the one spot on this earth where I could put down my own roots, feel as if I belonged and stay forever.

It was in this climate that the word "Tumut" surfaced again on my meditation walks with Sabina. I say again for I had seen it first in my early meditation in Canberra in the mid-1980s. Then I was surprised, nonplussed even, for although I knew the town well by reputation, I had never been there. Yet this word "Tumut" floated up out of nowhere and not just once but insistently. I talked to a close university friend. "Oh, it's a very beautiful place," he replied, "lovely water and magnificent trees, I have always thought I might retire there one day and write a book." Surfacing again in Stockholm it came with additional thoughts of building a beautiful garden and establishing a retreat for those people for whom life had been a bit rough, who wanted to drop out, and regroup for a while in a quiet, beautiful place.

So I started to talk slowly to Ian of his retirement. There were many imponderables: when would it be, where would we go, what would we do? I wondered, I said, if after more than thirty-three years travelling the world, living his career, he would now consider coming with me to live the life I now thought I wanted to live. I talked quietly of my meditation, of Tumut, a retreat cottage and the possibility of building a different Rosen practice, one where people stayed overnight after a session. The idea gradually took shape. He had been to Tumut, he said, and it seemed a nice place. He had been born in the country and had always thought he might like to try farming.

At first he thought he would like one further posting. I demurred; I was keen to go now, at once, anything to get away from these feelings. We agreed on a compromise, he would seek appointment as Australian Consul General in San Francisco for a period of three years; that way I could continue my Rosen work at its birthplace in the nearby Bay Area. The Department and the Minister agreed, plans were under way for us to move there towards the end of 1990 and then came a letter. A letter that set the course for the rest of our lives — a turning point. The Department was sorry, so it was said, but the position in San Francisco was required by the Prime Minister for a political appointee and was no longer available for Ian.

Then I was not the only one anxious to leave the Department. Ian was very angry. After a lifetime of faithful service, going without fuss wherever he had been sent, he felt he deserved better. And so the fateful decision to take early retirement after the Stockholm posting was taken. On 1 December 1991 Ian formally retired and we took possession of 160 acres of farming land and a comfortable house in the Goobragandra Valley on the banks of the Goobragandra River, just eighteen kilometres east of Tumut in southern New South Wales. "Binowee" in Flinders might have been sold when my mother moved to Melbourne, but it rose again from the ashes as "Binowee" on the banks of the Goobra.

We moved in with unprecedented amounts of luggage: sea luggage from Stockholm, furniture from store in Canberra, my mother's possessions from Melbourne, some of Ian's mother's possessions also from Melbourne. Amidst all this confusion two things stand out for me. My small three-year-old grand-daughter saying confidentially to one of the removalists, "Abba (her name for me) says she is never ever going to move again." Ian found in the new vegetable garden at 4pm, quietly planting beans and lettuces.

The Faces of Freedom

When I think of our life in Tumut the first word that comes to mind is *freedom* and this in all its facets and every aspect of our lives. First, and most obviously was freedom from the constraints imposed by living the life of a permanent officer of the Department of Foreign Affairs and Trade. Over the years this life had dictated where we lived, when we travelled and what we did most weekends. It was difficult to plan ahead and impossible to be absolutely certain about anything. Once posted, health, education, timing of leave and much of our free time were all to a great extent controlled by the demands of representing Australia abroad, and looking after visitors. To wake on those first mornings in Tumut knowing that we could do whatever we wanted whenever we wanted was heady stuff.

Simultaneously many of our previous financial limitations seemed to have vanished, largely perhaps because our four children had all finished their tertiary education. Now with Ian's superannuation and some funds from the estates of both our mothers we could do pretty much whatever we wanted. Since we were both relatively young and fit, health was also not a controlling factor. So in the outer aspects of our lives there seemed to be freedom aplenty.

Therefore in those early months of 1992, the first question was what exactly did we want to do now that we had arrived. This brought us to an often overlooked face of freedom, the necessity to choose, to make choices. Since nobody was telling us what to do, we had to choose for ourselves, although the fact that we had purchased farming land, would dictate some of our moves. In all fairness to our neighbours we would have to be responsible farmers, build fences, plant trees, spray blackberries, graze cattle or sheep to keep down other weeds and fire hazards and drench our animals to play our part in minimising disease. Clearly responsibility to the community in which we planned to live was another face of freedom.

Our neighbours offered advice on what would be easiest and most economically viable. Here was the necessity to make other choices, together with another face of freedom, responsibility — the choice itself would be our responsibility. We would have to live it and live with it. We would not be able to play the victim and blame others if it became apparent we had chosen poorly. This meant we should choose something we enjoyed doing and that required skills we had some hope of acquiring, so that we were not overly dependent on our neighbours. In the end we opted for a small herd of breeding cows (about twenty), a bull and a flock of about a hundred sheep. Later, feeling he should contribute usefully to the community, Ian chose to help with the local show, Landcare and the firebrigade.

With the farm under way, it was time to consider those other reasons that had brought us to Tumut — the establishment of the retreat and a beautiful garden. More freedom and more choices. What type of retreat were we planning? Would our guests live in the house with us? Would we build a retreat cottage, and if so, of what design? Slowly things fell into place. In my mother's papers, I found an article about the Goulburn Yurtworks that my mother had saved when Ian and I had been travelling in Outer Mongolia. We had loved the yurts we had seen there; now it appeared that here in Tumut we could have our own yurt constructed of wood.

Thus was born the idea of the "Yurt at Binowee", an idyllic retreat used by dozens of people in the ensuing years. Bushwalkers, meditators, birdwatchers, buddhists on silent retreat, stargazers, people coming to terms with death, divorce, retrenchment, cancer or any of the many blows life can inflict, all came and went telling us how much they had appreciated the quiet beauty we had to offer.

Although the Goobragandra Road divided the property, the house itself was right on the banks of the Goobragandra River. Sitting outside one day soon after our arrival, browsing through a book on landscaping, I read of the importance of a backdrop in good garden design. I looked up, no worry there. We had a most beautiful setting; the land sloped down from the house to the cheeky, bubbling river. The opposite bank rose up into a natural bush-covered hill under the blue sky above. As I saw it, my main problem would be to avoid detracting from the natural beauty with which we were surrounded.

Finally there was my Rosen life. Did I intend to establish a practice as a Rosen practitioner? If so where? In Tumut, in Canberra or possibly in Wagga Wagga, the largest town within ready reach of Tumut with a population of over 50,000 people and only an hour's drive away? Much freedom, more choices. After some hesitation a plan developed, I would work in Tumut if possible, but also travel to Canberra four days a month to develop a Rosen practice and a client base for the yurt. In fact developing a Rosen practice proved relatively easy. What became more difficult was to limit my numbers. This has been a continuing paradox in the development of Rosen Bodywork in Australia. Yes, we need publicity in order to promote the work, but, no, we can't have too much, for even now, ten years later, we lack sufficient practitioners to cope.[72]

Writing this now some ten years after the event, it sounds as though two carefree spirits made their choices and waved their wands. Not so. Weeks, months and, in the case of the garden, years went by as we planned and worked. Both of us were often simultaneously exhilarated by our exciting adventure and exhausted both by the unaccustomed physical exercise and the learning of so many new things. Frustration was always

---

[72] I have written of the choices involved in the decision to concentrate on writing and developing a Rosen practitioner training program separately, see, *The Scholar's Gown*, p. 188

close at hand both at the slow pace of life in the country and, particularly in my case, my own perceived inadequacies.

Enter another most important face of freedom — the ability to be free, or at least, less hassled by my perceived inadequacies, free from the restrictions I placed on myself. I sometimes used to wonder if I had been "set up" by the Universe, set up to choose to do something completely different from anything I had ever previously attempted, so that the challenge of not feeling inadequate would be continuous. It was easy to tell myself that I had done my Rosen training and learnt of those childhood incidents that had influenced the woman I had become. It was easy to say to myself that now I had the chance to move beyond those psychological constraints, to be free of fear of the unknown, free of bedevilling feelings of inadequacy, of being wrong, free to joyfully live this very beautiful life I had chosen.

It was very much more difficult, though, to actually live that way. Slowly, and with as much patience as I could muster, I had to apply what I had learnt to the living of my new life and allow myself to work my way through Marion's stages.[73] So there were endless opportunities for the use of the mirror of life and countless occasions to practise moving beyond limiting feelings. Would I ever reach the point where I could just flow with the current of my life, trusting that I was in the right place at the right time doing what was expected of me in the dance of my life? Self-acceptance and trust go hand in hand here, trusting the Universe, trusting myself; surely trust has to be another face of freedom.

So in the summer of 1992, with high hopes we began our new life in Tumut. The children and I thought Ian looked wonderful striding his acres in jeans, boots, akubra and his kelpie at heel.[74] He looked as if he had been born to the part. One of our new-found Tumut friends christened him "the squire", we all liked that. As for me, even if I did not blend into the landscape quite as easily as Ian, I had this quite beautiful feeling that I had come "home", come to rest in a place where I felt I belonged and could put down roots. When sadly and most unexpectedly about eight and a half years later we had to make the hardest choice of all, that of

---

[73] See *The Mirror of Life*, p. 153

[74] An akubra is a wide-brimmed typically Australian hat made of felt from pressed rabbit skins. A kelpie is an Australia sheep dog.

leaving Tumut, we both agreed those years had been the loveliest posting we had ever had.

Most of the letters to my imaginary friend that follow were written in our first few months in Tumut. I am clearly struggling with my role in the move and my capacity to live this very different life. "*He Came Oh So Still…*" on the other hand, was written when we had been in Tumut over a year, and reflects blessedly growing feelings of ease and tranquillity.

Snakes in the Grass

The Nix at Work[75]

Dear Friend,

Well, here it is, the first letter from Judith, farmer's wife. It is January 1992, and we have now been in our new home for a little over a month and are busily discovering all we don't know about life on the land. It's another leap in the dark, Friend, a huge one this time, away from Canberra, friends and the well-known fabric of Foreign Affair's life.

In due course, I think we will have to take a farming partner, one who has all the expertise and the correct equipment. Just at the moment we are struggling alone. I suppose it is hardly surprising that I feel anxious, close to panic, with my well-known feelings of fear of the unknown and not being able to cope, surfacing round me. Let's face it, farming life is absolutely unknown to me, although blessedly not quite so much so to Ian. Let's face it also we know absolutely no one in the town apart from the Estate Agent who sold us the property and some of our neighbours who have been very friendly. So here we are alone, just the two of us, struggling to pump our own drinking water from the river, control cattle, maintain electric fences and adjust to the inherent independence required for country living. Yes, I am sure our neighbours would help more frequently with some of these problems if we asked; but we feel we can't ask all the time. We do have to learn to do these things for ourselves.

Goobragandra Road divides our property in two. A couple of weeks ago we started our first major project, linking the electric fence from those two sections through a culvert under the road. The culvert itself, half filled with water, had heavily grassed verges sloping down steeply to swampy reedy patches outside its mouth on both sides of the road. Oh, how I hate that culvert; dining with the King at the Palace in Stockholm seems a lifetime away.

---

75 School and University friends call Ian "Nick"; some of my children are called "Nick" by some of their friends; a close and supportive group of my friends call me Mrs Nick. So when we were searching for a name for our farming partnership we chose "The Nix".

Ian needs my help, and I can hardly refuse him, since this entire move to Tumut and all it entails was my idea. Yet as I handled that cable along its journey to the culvert something inside me just freaked: I had butterflies in my stomach and seemed to be all a-tremble at least on the inside. At the time, since I was not wearing gumboots and my legs were very exposed, I told Ian I was frightened of snakes. Yet even as I spoke, I knew snakes were not really the problem for they hold little fear for me. Be that as it may, I am terrified to go near that culvert. Ingrid would say it has its hooks in my unconscious in a very big way. What is all this about?

A few days later while in Canberra for a wedding, I went to see Amy. "You look so tired, Judith," she said, "what is going on in your life?" Tears came, it was my old and faithful friend, I said, the move to Tumut was all just too much, I just couldn't handle it, couldn't cope. It seemed like a Foreign Affairs posting all over again. Overseas there would have been support staff at an embassy whose job it was to help us settle in, and on whom we could therefore rely without guilt. We talked then of needing to take things quietly, not trying to organise the whole house and farm in a matter of days or weeks, and of course, my old friend, trust — learning to trust, trust, trust. The inspiration for this whole move had surfaced in my meditation; therefore presumably the Universe would have a hand in the resolution of some of these seemingly insuperable problems.

Yet there was something else, I could feel it. "I have to help Ian put an electric cable through a culvert under a road," I murmured, "I simply don't understand the depth and intensity of my feelings of fear around it." There was a pause for a minute. "Can you give me an image of that fear," she said, "how do you see it?" Suddenly there I was in a long dark tunnel — the vagina — struggling, fighting to be born. It was dark, slimy and airless; the more I struggled, the worse the situation seemed to become. And fear was everywhere, I seemed to be all but engulfed, swallowed up in it. And with that fear there was pain, so much pain on the right side of my head. Suddenly I felt myself pulled, yanked, coughing and spluttering out into the light. Well, well, there it was, there was my explanation: Judith's birth, my birth being replayed nearly fifty-nine years later over a cable through a culvert, in an overall situation that was clearly one of re-birth.

That same afternoon I went to see the acupuncturist seeking help for a nasty pain in my right shoulder and up into the right side of my neck. Suggesting it was the gall bladder meridian, he talked of fats (of which I eat very little), and alcohol (my one small daily brandy seemed unlikely to be responsible). "The Chinese regard frustration as the emotional state connected to the gall bladder," he murmured quietly. Bingo, a bull's eye, the words were no sooner out of his mouth than I saw it. Frustration, of course, so very obvious, and for that reason, perhaps, unseen.

I have been locked in the process of re-birth at every level since we came to live in Tumut. And I am frustrated at every conceivable level: I am not physically fit enough, do not know what I should know about farming. I am too sensitive, not calm enough, not trusting enough. On and on I go endlessly whipping myself, frustrated because I am not good enough for this new life I have chosen, and unable to accept that I am as I am, that it is all right for me to be as I am, for that is how the Divine designed me to be for my small part in the play of life.

How often did my feelings, my stigmata as Jan called them, that I am not good enough, can't cope, my near obsessive need to be better, surface in my sessions with Ingrid? How often did she bring me back to the thief on the cross beside Jesus at the crucifixion to whom Jesus said he would see him in Heaven that night? There you are, she used to say. Just exactly as you are, no stress, no changing anything, no going anywhere, just exactly as you are, you are good enough. You don't have to be perfect; you only have to be yourself. If you try to be perfect you fail endlessly, and your perpetual state is one of frustration. Then the ego is constantly in pain because it always sees itself as inadequate, unable to cope, imperfect.

All of these insights brought a great sense of relief. Looking back I seemed to have been thrashing fruitlessly and frantically for months — probably ever since I left Sweden. It has been so hard at times to stay balanced and calm in such new waters with no real idea of where I am going. Ah, Friend, here we come to another piece of the puzzle — my near obsessive need to be able to see a pattern in my life. For me just to flow quite out of control in the waters of life seems to be well nigh impossible. Where is that trust? Heigh-ho, I need a little more compassion and tenderness for myself, perhaps, that I keep heaping such pain on myself.

And so we returned to Tumut to complete the linking of that jolly cable through the culvert. It was really hard for me, although easier with the gumboots we had purchased in Canberra. I shook; felt panicky and tears were close all day. There was only one real surprise: when Ian was mattocking a particularly obstinate patch of weeds suddenly, involuntarily, I flinched, cringed and threw up my hands to protect my head. Simultaneously I saw-felt the cruel bite of the forceps on that tiny baby's frail skull, my skull, as I was born. It was an extraordinary experience, a Rosen session beside a country road in rural Australia, bringing to the fore all the feelings I had had at my birth and described to Amy.

All in all it took five long hours finally to connect the cable through the culvert. I don't remember when I was last so exhausted. Perhaps being born, re-born effects one like that! Alone and unaided we had done it. We tottered back to the house and had a drink to celebrate. The Nix work on the farm; perhaps we would make farmers after all…

As I write, Friend, I realise this letter seems hard on our farming neighbours who on our arrival gave much of the support for which country people are renowned and which we appreciated greatly. However, we felt rightly, I am sure, that we couldn't continually rely on their goodwill to make our dream come true.[76] We had to do it ourselves and we did.

Wish me luck, Friend, I certainly need all the help and support I can find at the moment.

---

[76] Within a few months we resolved this problem by forming a small informal joint venture with one of our experienced farming neighbours.

Whose Body?

Hello Friend,

What is it I wonder that is struggling to come up from my unconscious today, that needs a letter to you to bring it forth? That title selected itself as soon as I sat down to write. *Whose Body?* I wonder what I need to say about that?

If I start with the physical, as I used to do when I wrote in Sweden, then I know that my body has undergone considerable change since we arrived in Tumut, and is feeling very stressed as a result. It is fitter with all the planting, painting and cleaning up. It is also quite abominably tired at the moment; not the sort of fatigue that needs sleep, or even bed rest; but one which craves just to be left alone. The painter, a most helpful woman, asked me to decide a question about stains last evening. I heard myself say to her, "I'll tell you in the morning, I am just too tired to decide anything more tonight."

As we both know I have driven my body on and on — the move from Sweden to Tumut, the getting on top of country life, the beginning of our garden and now the alterations and renovations to the house. "Binowee" is my dream, my lifetime's piece of creative work.

In the language of the unconscious a house is symbolic of many different things — the psyche, the soul, and also in some literature, the human body. Since I have been straining my body and remaking my house I could ask what have I been doing to my psyche?

Ingrid used to tell me time and again in Sweden that my outer life was always a reflection of my inner, what I call the mirror of life. So my answer to my question must be along the lines that I have been refashioning my psyche and very possibly straining as I went. There is some imp in me, you know, which drives me on. I know now, so very well, that I don't have to strain, there is no need. How many times have I now experienced that things happen as and when they are supposed to? No earlier no later. If that is so, and my mind knows that it is, then straining is a waste, a total, absolute waste of time. And yet I strain; Ian is out in the paddocks straining too. God in heaven what drives us all?

Our ego, that's what it must be. My sense that I, Judith Nicholson, driving myself on in my ageing body, I am responsible for my life, my project, the fulfillment of my dreams. Ah, as I write I see something else: I am also driven by my age. I am fifty-nine, now finally, after all these years waiting and helping others, I have my chance to live my life, and as I experience it, there is so little time left. I will soon become older, frailer and eventually die. So, on we go, says my ego, faster, faster, more, more!

Heavens, Friend, it is so still today. For the first time I am sitting at my desk in its appointed place, in an east-facing nook, looking up the Goobragandra Valley. The world sparkles in the winter sun this afternoon. Nothing moves and I am here, in my appointed place. My ego is housed in my body and together we are housed in my jewel-like "Binowee". This is a beautiful place; it is a privilege to be able to live here, a sacred trust to be custodian of such a treasured place.

Did I, Judith Nicholson, bring this about? Did I arrange for this house to come on the market just as we left Sweden? Did I bring myself an honest, friendly, estate agent/stock agent to help us become established? Did I bring us a professional farming partner, a thoughtful, helpful builder, a delightful house painter and Rosen Method support in Tumut of all places? Did I? Did I? **NO**

The only possible answer is **No**. There is no conceivable way I could have achieved all this on my own. At every stage, at every point another piece of the puzzle slides gently into place. If I can only keep my ego out of it there is no need to strain, none at all. All I need to do is to remind myself that I, Judith Nicholson, am part of the Divine Plan. The Plan involves me as some sort of custodian of this body, being in this place, at this time, that's all.

Idling

Floating gently with the beauty of the moment

Dear Friend,

Idling, a curious thought isn't it, in this busy world where most people don't feel comfortable with themselves unless they can tell you how "buuuusy" they are. Right now, I am suffering at the hands of busy people. Recently arrived in Tumut, feeling a bit anxious and in need of support, I have asked friends of long-standing to visit me in Tumut, or at least lunch with me on my visits to Canberra. "Oh I can't, I'm sorry, I'm too busy, so very busy," has been the reply, followed by a long list of more important things they feel they must do. Unnerved and unsettled as I have been by Ian's retirement and our move to live here, I have felt rejected and valueless as I faced the hard fact that they were too busy to have time for me.

Then the words *idle, idling*, began to surface in my meditation with such intensity of feeling as to bring tears to my eyes. I saw them first in contrast to the word "busy". Born and raised in a family strongly influenced by the Protestant work ethic, I too have previously felt it almost sinful not to be busy; yet now, my life is keeping me away from busy people and my meditation is insisting the word idle has a place in my life. Surely in the midst of one of the more daring ventures of my life, I am not supposed to be sitting with hands folded in my lap gazing into space?

Then one night recently an intuition floated up. We say engines idle, an additional meaning to the word. What do I mean, though, if I say my car engine, the only engine I know well, is idling? I checked in the dictionary: *idle, to operate, usually at minimum speed, while the transmission is disengaged*. So if I say my car engine is idling, I mean that the motor has been started, is running quietly, smoothly, waiting for me to sit in the seat, belt up and move off — to engage the transmission.

Idling then is not only the opposite of busy; it is also a state of mind when one is quietly watching and waiting, alert, ready to step out as soon as the moment is right. Long experience has taught me this is the state of mind in which my unconscious makes itself heard. I now realise I was idling as I walked quietly with Sabina in those beautiful Swedish forests. My mind was often quiet, flat, not pulled by a thousand thoughts about this and that. In that space there was time for my unconscious to make itself heard, to pop up as it were and say, "Oh, by the way, have you considered such and such?"

It is a distrustful ego that strains, pushing and pulling this way and that, allowing us little peace. The Yogis talk of attempting to live in and trust the moment, not fretting about what might have been — the "if onlys" of one's life, nor racing off into the future — the "what ifs". If while doing one thing, they suggest, my mind is anxiously swinging back and forth, then I am not truly focussed on each minute of my life, not actually living my life. If my mind was able to live that way and a very big if it is, then it would be idling in my new meaning of the word and I would have peace and tranquillity. In fact I would be serene. My pen stills as I write that word, *serene*. Ever since I was a very young teenager I have wanted for two things — wisdom and serenity — well, well...

Over the years, I had walked quietly in many beautiful places — along rivers, through forests, around lakes. As I walked, I left behind the past and did not look to the future. I floated as it were, quietly, gently, with the beauty of the moment. I idled...

I sit at my desk looking up my beautiful valley. So much has been done, yes, and there would be other things to do tomorrow, next week, next month. But today the sun shines, the newborn lambs cavort with their mothers, the yellow wattles gleam.

And so, I idle, quietly in the beauty of this moment.

Who am I?

Dear Friend,

An identity crisis is what I seem to be having at this moment. Who the hell am I? After all these years of bodywork and meditation, delving into myself, spreading out all the pieces I could lay my hands on, both good and bad, what do we actually know about me?

My passion for bodywork tells us something — that I am enthusiastic, passionate about the tasks I undertake. Old Grandfather Wyatt used to boom out, "If a job's worth doing, it's worth doing well." He must have engraved that on my heart. All my adult life I have driven myself, my family and my colleagues, forcing on all the necessity of doing the job well.

Working with Ingrid in Sweden, I came to accept intellectually that I was a perfectionist and, with much coaching from her, that I need not be perfect to be a part of the Divine. From time to time I do feel that self-acceptance now. I do feel that wondrous freedom to be just exactly as I am, doing just exactly what I am supposed to be doing. The freedom to be Judith Nicholson, living at "Binowee", here in Tumut, without the need to change a single thing. Then something happens, I react sharply, or else I am in unexplained physical pain. Immediately, despite all Ingrid's wise counsel, my mind, both conscious and unconscious, leaps to tell me that this is healing, a release of negative energy that is necessary that I may be accepted as part of the Divine.

Perhaps I should now be more specific. I have had chronic pain down the right side of my head now for the last couple of years. It comes and goes, but at its worst it is nasty. Ingrid and I worked with it many times. That area was hurt by the forceps at my birth. So we looked at my fears and feelings of abandonment.[77] Recently I wrote to her saying my head was still bothering me. In her reply she suggests there may be something deeper that we didn't find initially, and wonders if

---

77 See *Birthday*, p. 110

there are feelings of panic and frustration when the pain returns.

Now when we looked at my birth, as I felt it I became stuck because of my mother's fears, and we agreed I took on a "fear of the unknown", both hers and mine. Last night I re-lived that experience, relived those feelings of being trapped, helpless, and powerless to move myself from that situation unaided. Beneath all of those feelings I found one we missed before, a confusing diabolic blend of panic and frustration. How could I move, who would help me move, what was going to happen to me? Now if I return to the present, how many times since I came to live here in the country have I felt helpless, inadequate, waiting for someone to "pull me out"? Countless would have to be the answer. It is all so new, demands so many skills, so much physical strength that I don't appear to have. No wonder I am close to panic, no wonder I am so frustrated and my self-confidence is shaky. Little wonder my head thumps so much.

This morning I have stood on the edge of that panic. It seems to be at the "bottom of my being", down in the depths somewhere. I approach it on tiptoe; I can feel myself quivering, twitching, like a horse or a dog, anxious to flee danger. I have been there wondering do I need to touch this feeling, release it from my body? Or, is it enough simply to know of its presence and feel its power?

It seems, at least at the moment, that this latter is sufficient. I need to understand that a powerful driving force is the fear of panic. This I now realise, is a fundamental part of my patterning. This is the Judith who has sought knowledge from every source, to understand, and thus learned many languages; who has aimed to be competent, efficient, administratively on top of her life, anything rather than have her life on top of her. This way I have at least had a modicum of control, some pattern or structure in my life and can keep the panic at bay. Yes, but while I do this, I leave very little room in my life for trust. Ah me, trust, trust, one of the most difficult parts of my spiritual journey. Sometimes I think I must be the original doubting Thomas.

So, to return to my heading, who am I? One answer is that I am an ego-based person, Judith Nicholson, who has the attributes I have just listed — a passion, a desire for perfection, who feels helpless, powerless, fearful, and panicky and yes frustrated, so dreadfully frustrated that she is unable to trust. What haven't I listed? Why, the desire for love. To be able to give love, to receive love, "to be" love in some way.

So, why should this be surfacing from my unconscious at this time? And why the depth of frustration? From where I stand now I can see it all. I can see the Judith Nicholson I have lived with all these years, all her hopes and all her fears. But now at this time, I am beginning to see another Judith, the one whose adventures on her spiritual path have been told in her letters and reflections. I am beginning to know her well, know that she is lovely. She is warm, passionate, loving, wise, comforting, full of fun, full of joy. She burns with a passionate desire to live this wonderful life she has been offered to the fullest possible extent. She wants to dance for the very joy of living.

And what stands in her way? Those old patterns of her mind, of course. Those worn out old tracks on an overused gramophone record still cackling on about fear, inadequacy, panic and mistrust. As I paused for thought here, a lovely image came to mind. Recently I bought a new stylus for our very old gramophone. Yesterday as I did the ironing, I listened to some of my old and most favourite records. They had been transformed.

Is it possible a new stylus is coming into my life, transforming my old records, allowing me to hear my favourite music at its most beautiful, smoothing out the wrinkles, removing the frustrations? And the name of the stylus? It would have to be trust, Friend, wouldn't it? The name of the game, trust, trust. I can't yet write that this other Judith is a trusting person; but I can at least say she is much more trusting than she used to be.

Let me return to my original question, who am I? Well, first of all I am an ego-based Judith, we all know that. Secondly, we seem to have a person who used to feel one way and is now moving towards a group of new feelings. Two of these deserve special mention. To be be-loved, that wondrous, free, joyous feeling of a person who is loved just exactly as she is. Finally, to feel a small unique part of the Divine World. This is a relatively new feeling for me. I imagine every person experiences it in his or her own particular way. For me, it seems to bring a freedom, a wonderful freedom just to be myself, and then a warmth, a vibrancy, love, joy and compassion.

So, that's who I am, Friend, I am Judith, just Judith, small, unique and my own special part of the Divine...

The Scholar's Gown

In July 1995, I set out to find about twenty interested participants for the first Introductory Workshops for Rosen Method Bodywork in Australia. The response was slow until the last minute. Then suddenly, as a result of a half page feature story in the *Canberra Times* and an interview on ABC radio in Canberra, the phone rang constantly and I had my numbers.

Workshops completed, the phone continued to ring. The *Canberra Times* article had struck a cord with many people. Suddenly the Yurt was heavily booked, I was giving my maximum numbers of sessions each week, and the phone was still ringing insistently; people wanted to see me to talk of and experience the body-mind connection.

After the long training in Sweden, my three years practising in Australia alone, you would have thought I would have been delighted, excited at the prospect of a flourishing Rosen practice. Not a bit of it! I could feel the resistance in myself as I spoke to people on the phone. I knew, even if my callers didn't, that the usual welcoming warmth was missing from my voice. What on earth was this about?

I spoke to Ian. I was bowled over, I said, confused, uncertain what to do. I hadn't expected such a response. "Oh," he replied, "it is exactly what I expected would happen; I thought this was what you wanted, I thought you would be happy." Well I wasn't happy, that much was clear, even if my other reactions were shrouded in confusion.

A few weeks later, I talked quietly with Amy. She asked about the public reaction to all the recent Rosen publicity and how I was finding my new life. My resistance to the lack of freedom in my life surfaced immediately. "I feel trapped," I said, "and I hate it, people keep ringing wanting sessions; I have no time for myself, no time to manoeuvre." She talked quietly of the life of a "healer': the need to care for myself, to set boundaries. I could feel my resistance growing as she talked; something was wrong, this wasn't me.

Suddenly I saw that I didn't want to be a "healer". I said so clearly. We were both surprised. After I started meditating and became aware of the warm healing energy in my hands, we had both assumed I would use it in some way. But, "NO," said my intuition firmly and clearly, "that is not what I am about." It was as if out shopping for clothes I had said to a shop assistant brooking no discussion, "I do not want that gown, the blue gown of healing, it doesn't fit correctly, doesn't really suit me."

Amy and I talked then of teaching at which I had spent much of my adult life: teaching English in the US language school on a posting to Phnom Penh, third grade in the British Primary School on that same posting, French for the *Alliance Francaise* in Canberra, and my more formal career as a University law lecturer. It had been a fair assumption that I would be involved in teaching Rosen Bodywork in Australia. "Not so," said my intuition, again loudly and clearly: "writing, talking of bodywork, yes, but teaching as a qualified teacher in a regular training program, no." So, no black teacher's gown either.

The faces of freedom lurked unspoken as we talked. Having established my Rosen practice both in Canberra and at Tumut, set in motion the first steps for an Australian Rosen practitioner training program, it now appeared I had other choices to make. I was bothered by questions of selfishness. How was I to justify myself, I asked Amy, not helping, not teaching, when there was a need, and I had the skills; see the good girl lurking.[78] We talked then of my own needs, my obligation to consider

---

78 And this despite my brush with breast cancer which had established that I needed to pay greater attention to "nourishing myself", see *A Cancer Saga*, p. 201

these, doing only those things that coincided with them. All right, but what were my needs? As I groped towards an answer with Amy, writing became the key. I felt as if I was being driven to write; everything else was of less importance. It seemed I needed experience with clients and some teaching but of themselves they were not my *raison d'etre*; rather a means to gain the necessary experience for my writing.

Later that same day, I had a "road to Damascus encounter", such was the intensity of my intuition. The gown I wanted was a scholar's gown, the red gown awarded to Ph.D. graduates of some universities. For me the word scholar has long carried a deep emotional intensity. I was delighted once to find in a dictionary that it had the dual meaning of pupil, or disciple with a master, and one who is learned. I love that conjunction of meaning; one is both learning and learned. The day of that encounter, I realised I had always wanted to be a "scholar" and had been endlessly frustrated unconsciously by the good girl roles of family and Foreign Affairs. No wonder I was resistant, contrary and confused with these phone calls from prospective clients. They were pulling me away yet again from my possible scholar's life.

This time the intuition was clear and unequivocal: in some way I wanted to be a scholar in the remainder of my life. I might work as a bodyworker, or as an assistant teacher; but only that I might add more insight and more depth to my own knowledge. During these last ten years, while seeking meaning for my own life, I had been exploring the body-mind-spirit connection within my own body. Now it seemed my own unique creative spark and the joy it could bring, lay in the writing of this journey.

Why this emphasis on the scholar and scholarship, though? Why do these words carry such power for me? Lying in bed, floating with ideas of scholars and scholarship, I thought of the few genuine scholars I knew. What set them apart from other people? What were they showing me? A word floated "free". The scholars I knew seemed to be free, inspired by the pursuit of knowledge for its own sake rather than the status or money it might bring. Moreover, despite undoubted learning, their minds were free. They had openness, a curiosity, a willingness to take a fresh idea, play with it, toss it about, see where it might lead. I loved the freedom to draw and re-draw my own pattern in the desert sands. This freedom though, has to be combined with a rigorous personal integrity, otherwise your scholar becomes a charlatan, chasing ideas in the wind; manipulating them for his or her own ends.

Later as I quietly talked to Jennifer of my new found scholar and where she fitted into my life, another piece of the puzzle fell into place. We agreed that now I had finally identified my own needs for my own life, it would be possible for me to set boundaries without guilt: to say quietly and firmly, "I am sorry I am not seeing new clients at the moment, I am writing a book about the bodywork." This, as it turned out, was easier said than done: good girls die a hard death, still it was a start. At least I had chosen my gown.

Nowadays emphasis is placed on proof by an outside, allegedly objective measurement. A doctor once said to me, "You can't prove the body-mind connection even in generalisations about stress." No I can't. Neither can he. We are dealing in possibilities, which in time may grow into probabilities and ultimately into hard scientific fact. However, in the realm of feelings and spirit, scientific proof may always be elusive, and in any event unnecessary. My clients, students and I, none of us need an instrument to tell us there is a relationship between our feelings and the ease or lack of ease in our bodies, we know. Our friends and families don't need scientific proof either. They look at our faces, notice our changed attitudes and see the connection and ensuing transformation for themselves.

Years ago bodywork came from nowhere and grabbed me, I have tried to follow its wisdom ever since. When offered the choice I chose to wear the red gown of the scholar, seeking meaning and understanding with an open, unbiased mind, following ideas as they presented themselves to me, playing with them, rejecting some, retaining others, modifying, testing as I went. Now it seems I belong to no one school of thought, yet I have built a myth or a story of my life and its purpose that feels good to me.

'He came oh so still,
That His mother was,
As dew in April
That lyeth on the grass.'

Dear Friend,

Hello, I have my fingers crossed for a restful and refreshing summer. Last year seemed a bit much all round. That's one of the reasons I am drawn to the lyric in the heading. Stillness. The shining, shimmering peace of dew on the grass early on a spring morning (in the Europe of the lyric, that is). I don't know the origin of that lyric. In my last year at school, the twelve voice Madrigal Group of which I was a member, made a recording of Benjamin Britten's Ceremony of Carols. The verse was there, a haunting soprano solo. It gripped me then as it does to this day.

So, what am I on about this morning? Something way out to judge by my heading. In the proverbial nutshell, birth is the word. It's all around me, reflecting to me where I am, as Ingrid would have said.[79] All our children were here at "Binowee" for Christmas; two new grandchildren expected September — October. The first of the Binowee babies. A pretty fertile spot, perhaps.

In my own case it is hardly birth I am looking at, not at my age. Although if I spent some effort last year working through the various feelings involved in my own birth. There seemed to be a number of "nasties" there, and they needed to come up to the light.

If I pause, I can see a beautiful image that has appeared these last couple of nights. I am a woman, a youngish woman, and I glow with vitality, it is a significant thing about me, vitality, vibrancy. It is as if I am Life itself. I imagine I have just given birth to a tiny, beautifully formed baby daughter. I am quiet in my own bed, here in my beautiful bedroom at "Binowee". Beautiful because it is light, airy, sunny and looks out on three sides; south to the river, east up the valley to the

[79] See *The Mirror of Life*, p. 153

rising sun, and north to the ring of protective hills behind.

There are three people in the bed in my image: the mother, the father and the baby daughter. The father is in the centre, in his role as protector of the small flock. He holds his baby daughter cradled in his left arm. The mother lies curled into his right side, his arm around her too, her hand fondling the toes of the baby. A soft white light tinged with the palest blue shimmers around this trio. No-thing, no-body moves. There is no need. They are at one with themselves, with each other and with all things with-in and with-out the house. As one — peace, absolute peace. As if One.

And the feelings? In the father there seems to be veneration that any woman would love, could love, could be so trusting, so open, so out of control, that she would/could let her body conceive, carry and give birth to their, his child. There is veneration, awe and deep down a living bubble of joy. Suddenly he feels so happy, so very happy, he wants to laugh, run, shout for joy. In the stillness a slow sure smile lights his face.

But what of the mother? I pause again here, I am looking at an image of myself. What do I feel as I lie quietly, at rest in my bed? A feeling comes flooding in, not the one I expected, actually; but it is very strong and it will not be denied. Relief, such an overwhelming sense of relief, of release from the burdens of a job to be done and now done; and of satisfaction also, from the knowledge that t'were well done. As I look on from the outside, I feel there ought to be other feelings: gratitude for the father who has stayed, supported and protected through all the ups and downs, mood swings, vagaries, fears, joys that make up any process of giving birth; a deep and abiding trust in life itself that brings all this about; love and joy itself. Surely, I say, all these are present, they must be. In time the image in the bed replies, in time they will be. Now there is relief and this wondrous feeling of peace — nothing more.

The small baby, what of her? She is the centre, the focal point of all of this. Look where she is lying now. The father has stirred, shifted her to his right arm; the mother moves, kisses the baby gently on the head, takes her and places her cradled gently between her two parents. I look again at the scene in the bed. What does she feel, the baby? She feels relief also; being born is a tumultuous process. Now she feels the quiet, the warmth, the peace, the rock-like loving comfort of the father, the flowing sustaining love of the mother. As she lies a bubble floats to the surface of her mind, breaks. Suddenly she feels she is alive, feels life itself. It pulses through her, quietly at first then more strongly, more insistently. This is Life, this is where she has always wanted to be, right here in the midst of this glorious wonderful thing called Life. The beginnings of a smile flit across her face; she drifts gently off to sleep.

So I am on about birth, the birth of a child, the rebirth of an adult. Birth with its mixed bag of feelings; birth and rebirth together the corner stones of Life.

The Heart's Wisdom

In all my Rosen training the emphasis was on listening to my body, learning to hear its subtle nuances as my breath changed, a muscle fluttered and my body vibrated for a split second responding to a phrase that was powerful for it. Along with many of my fellow students, I found that to vibrate with such inner knowing was different from knowing something intellectually with my conscious mind. It seemed that this bodily inner knowing first came into consciousness as a deeply held, powerful feeling, and as such, was not easily swept away by later thought, logic or commonsense. The heart's wisdom…

In the latter part of my Rosen training as I moved beyond experiencing incidents repressed during my childhood, I entered new unconscious territory, a land of symbolic imagery, of feelings I had never imagined existed. This was a land of exquisite beauty, of creativity, the white rose, the little demons, a little mermaid and the dancer within — a land of magic and mystery, the heart's wisdom again, only this time from another place along the path.

Initially Ingrid and I chose to describe experiences such as the dancer within, for example, in the language of the Yogis, talking in terms of past life experiences, re-incarnation, karma or individual bondage and the goal of self-realisation. These ideas I had first met in 1972-73 when Ian and I did a course on Indian culture while living in New Delhi. Later I attended seminars on the *Bhagavad-Gita* — one of India's great spiritual writings — and learnt the Hindu view that we all live more than once — re-incarnation — and that in some way we carry the fruits of one life forward into future ones — karma. This was an intellectual exercise: something I did to broaden my general knowledge and help me understand the community in which I was living. I was neither shocked nor attracted by it.

Then in 1985 when I first went to see Amy, she talked to me in an Eastern or Hindu context and these ideas arose again. This time, to my own surprise, I found I simply accepted the doctrine of re-incarnation as being so axiomatic and obvious as hardly to need explanation. Neither did I have trouble with the concept of karma — that our previous living might affect our current circumstances in some way — although the purpose of it and how it could be said to operate I found to be vexed questions.

Meanwhile, in my own reading of the Jungian writers, I had seen imagery such as that described in *The Little Demons* or *The Dancer Within* discussed in the psychological language of archetypes from the collective unconscious assisting the psyche on its voyage of individuation — the voyage of each individual psyche towards its unique destiny. Again I had no philosophical difficulties with this explanation, although at times as a lay reader I found the writing dense and difficult. It was also clear from my reading that the Jungians would interpret my experiences such as *The White Rose* and *The Little Mermaid* by searching for a universally accepted meaning for such symbols.

Yet, for all the intellectual interest of these philosophical speculations of expert theoreticians, I gradually reached a point where the living breathing feelings themselves that accompanied my imagery became more important than any discussion about their source. The words used by others to describe my journey began to seem largely irrelevant, for the feelings themselves were of such breath-taking, indescribable beauty. How could I analyse the vitality and vibrancy — the face of creativity — which I experienced during *Digging for Joy*: the rollicking unbelievably heady feelings of freedom flowing from *The Little Mermaid*: the deep peace that flows from feeling be-loved, a consequence of *The White Rose*: the joy that came from seeing another view of myself, living myself, just being myself, dancing the dance of my own life which was one of the consequences of *The Dancer Within*. Here was a veritable treasure trove of feelings. The land of the heart's wisdom...

Then I remembered how, when I first went to see Amy, I would ask her if I could borrow a book about this or that. Smiling, she would reply well, yes of course I could, but that in due course I would use books less, as I came to find my own wisdom. At the time I found this most unlikely: Judith not read a book about something, impossible. Yet, so it has been. Over the years I have grown to use books less and less and, with much help from Ingrid in Sweden, and later from Jennifer on my return to Australia, I have come to treat this in depth imagery as a message from my unconscious which, as a part of my total psyche, offers what help it can in any situation. The heart's wisdom, my heart's wisdom...

For all their beauty, these new feelings were uncharted territory. Just how free was free? Just where did unconditional love end, or did it? My first steps in this new territory were hesitant, unsure; I lost my footing over and over again. "When you first experience new feelings," Ingrid would say, "you find one firm footing and then, as you move forward, there are boggy, marshy patches where you feel uncertain, slip, sink into the mud and lose your way again." Then she would add, using one of her favourite words, "It is as if you are walking through a *quagmire*, go quietly, take it gently, be very patient with yourself, it takes time, much time to learn to handle new feelings and integrate them into your being." And so we continued our sessions and she helped me unravel my insights.

It was not until 1994, after my return to Australia, that I found a framework of my own in which to place this beautiful interaction with my unconscious. A long-time admirer of Dorothy L. Sayers and her fictional detective, Lord Peter Wimsey, I came across and bought a collection of her writings hoping for some insights into his creation.[80] Thus I unexpectedly came across Sayers' analysis of the creative writing process. First, the creative idea which an author has, that which will make the writing unique, a largely unknown, but nonetheless powerful yardstick carried basically in the unconscious, against which each thought, word, sentence and part of the piece is measured. Secondly, the germination, bringing into existence of that idea — the actual writing of the piece. And thirdly, the power that is generated by the written piece among its readers.

Even more surprising was to see Sayers equate each part of that creative writing process to one figure of the Christian Trinity. God, an idea that we most of us carry, consciously or unconsciously, however we choose to express it, some powerful yet largely unconscious yardstick against which we seek to measure the meaning of our lives. Secondly, the bringing into existence of that idea as we exercise choices at the crossroads of our lives, the incarnation — Christ. Thirdly, the power generated by that idea as we live the book of our lives — The Holy Spirit. I was greatly attracted both by the simplicity and the beauty of this analysis. It was almost as if Sayers herself was in the room talking and I was replying, "Yes, yes that's how I feel it must be for me."

As is the way with all ideas, I then took Sayers' writings, played with them on my walks and made them my own. Was it possible, I wondered, that I have one major creative challenge in this life — to live the life of Judith to the best of my ability. Am I, then, as I travel through life, unconsciously testing each of my moments of choice against this yardstick; and then as I live the book of my life, am I inevitably influencing those around me as I go? "Yes," my intuition said, "yes, that's a good way to describe how the process works for you." And the in-depth imagery then, is a part of that creative process helping me as I make choices at each step through Ingrid's quagmire. The Heart's Wisdom...

And my dancer, how does she fit in here? One thing was clear from the beginning; she was personal, private and intimate, belonging solely in my inner life, bringing healing feelings that I needed to have about **me**. Thus she helped me overcome those diabolical feelings of a lack of self-

80 Ann Loades, *Dorothy L. Sayers: Spiritual Writings*, SPKC, Great Britain, 1993, pp. 63-69

worth which lie behind a fear of rejection — the feelings of being second rate, inadequate, never good enough, never able to cope, of which I had become conscious during my early training. However, my intuition said, she has nothing to do with how others might choose to see me, their views are not part of my unconscious life. Slowly I realised she was telling me I was dancing to the music of my life, an endless dance in which I must never falter though the dance be quiet, riotous, happy, sad, joyful or tragic.

Finally I glimpsed her as a manifestation of the Divine, the Divine in me, my own personal incarnation of the Divine. Not for me, apparently the mystical "God within" of the Christian texts, nor the incarnation of the Guru of the Eastern mystics, to neither of whom could my ever practical, non-abstract twentieth-first century mind relate. Instead my unconscious floated the image of a woman, full of the love and the joy of dance, a woman for whom I had a great natural empathy. My dancer, The Dancer Within…ah the beauty and the magic of that.

PART VII

A Cancer Saga

Cancer, 1. a malignant and invasive
growth or tumour,...
2. any evil condition or thing
that spreads destructively [...]

Macquarie Dictionary

What we observe is not nature itself,
but nature exposed to our method of questioning.

Werner Karl Heisenberg

Black Thursday

B*reast cancer and betrayal*, the two b's of Thursday 29 July 1993, the day on which I was asked by the technician who had given me a mammogram in Canberra, to wait as the radiologist wished to discuss the results with me. The day on which I heard him say that there was a growth in my left breast which was of a shape normally associated with cancer. It was therefore essential, he said, that I return to Tumut immediately to discuss these results with my general practitioner and make arrangements for the further necessary tests. A day on which my life seemed to grind to a halt and my knees felt as if they would buckle under me.

By July 1993 we had been in Tumut for just over eighteen months. Having formed a partnership with an experienced local farmer, many of our initial problems around the farm had slowly been resolved. We were in the final stages of building the yurt; I had in fact been helping the painter with the oiling of the interior the previous week. We expected to be able to have our first visitors in a month or so. My Rosen practice in Canberra was developing steadily. I had enough clients for each of my visits; as one left another came forward.

The garden, too, was progressing well. The previous year an avenue of thirty-five pin oaks had been planted down the drive. Over a hundred agapanthus now bordered the edge of the lower drive as it swept towards the house. A hedge of Australian native shrubs had been planted near the vegetable garden, both to provide protection from the wind and a habitat for such birds as might prey on the bugs that were attacking the vegetables. Finally, on this same visit to Canberra, I was to collect eighty-five rugosa roses for a thick prickly hedge to protect the garden from marauding cattle. A big family celebration was organised for the middle of August. We planned a happy time, celebrating my sixtieth birthday, christening the yurt and planting roses.

And now this. If I looked back I had had my intuitions, my dream if you like, from my meditation. I had followed it to the best of my ability, gone with Ian to develop it in Tumut and now, instead of the life I had envisaged, there was the likelihood — soon to be the reality — of breast cancer. Among the many painful feelings, one stood out in those early days — betrayal. Like many, many other experiencing cancer, I was bitter and deeply hurt, at what God, the Universe, The Divine, Fate, whatever word you like to use, had "done to me".

The next couple of weeks were an agony of indecision as we waited for the results of the tests that finally established a small malignant tumour in my left breast just above the nipple. Then we were once again in a world of choice; tough choices this time about possible treatments that might well effect my health and life expectancy. The following four months were a time of surgery and radiation therapy involving five days a week in Canberra, interspersed with weekends back in Tumut. During all this time I was strongly and lovingly supported by family and close friends. There were cards, phone calls, books, flowers, cups of coffee, quiet chats and, to my great delight, the loan of a house to use during my five-day long visits to Canberra each week for radiation therapy. It was almost as if the Universe were saying, "look you do have to have this cancer, and I am really sorry about that, but I will make it as easy for you as I possibly can."

Thursday 29 July 1993 was black indeed; the months of August to December were grey and grim. In fact it was not until the middle of 1994 that I felt sufficiently recovered to take up the many threads of my life again.

The following letters to my friend, written during that period, in no way detract from all the other support I was receiving. Rather they were a continuation of a well established habit in which, by exploring freely and tentatively the reflections from the mirror of my life, both psychological and spiritual, I steadied myself, and sought to understand what was happening to me on my unconscious travels, without fear of judgment or rejection.

Freaking Away

Dear Friend,

It is a cold, wet, winter's day on the Goobragandra. Heavens, when it rains in this part of the world it just teems. I am comforted by the fact that in many parts of the world rain is regarded as very auspicious. May it prove to be so.

Why the heading "freaking away", and why am I in need of auspicious omens? A lump, that's why; a nasty little lump on my left breast that showed up on a mammogram nearly two weeks ago. I have read the literature by now; nine out of ten lumps are benign, are not malignant, not cancer. So why am I freaking? Because mine is not a highly recommended shape: it is star-shaped and therefore, according to the radiologist's report, is quite probably malignant.

I wonder — can I write about this? I would dearly love to be able to, if only to steady myself. For never, ever, have I felt the skids under me to the extent that they have been these last two weeks. And this in itself is irrational. I know that, and yet, and yet... What on earth is it about the possibility of cancer of the breast that gives me this incredibly awful feeling? I can't face it, can't accept it, this can't be me; I must move, get away from my body, escape somehow from all the medical ho-ha. This is why I say I freak, I freak away. No, no, I cry, this can't, this mustn't be, me. And yet, it is. I have to accept it, stay with it, stay in this body and go through whatever my body requires.

There are two aspects to this. I have seen the second only as I wrote that last paragraph. The first is being totally out of control. I saw that almost immediately. The second must be acceptance. I have no option. I have to stand still, accept my lump, and accept whatever consequences it may bring.

Let me be more specific: the lump is small and near the surface. There is virtually no possibility that, even if malignant, I have terminal cancer. So we shouldn't be, and aren't, talking of fear of death. The first thing to surface though was such a terror of losing my left breast, the full mastectomy. I wonder about this: where does this feeling come from? Why is it so strong? Again the surgeon says he can see no real possibility of this; the removal of the lump itself should be sufficient — a lumpectomy. I have, though, made him note that I have consented only to the removal of the lump. If he thinks he needs to remove my breast then we have to discuss that further, even if that means I will have to have further surgery. I found I simply could not, would not, face any uncertainty as to the whereabouts of my left breast as I surfaced from the anaesthetic.

There is even more to it than that. Even the thought that someone is going to slice into my left breast with a scalpel can send me shivering and sobbing. What do we have here? I have faced other surgery with reasonable equanimity. Not this one.

I wonder. Am I replaying, out of the depths of my unconscious, myself as a tiny newborn baby whose nipples had to be lanced because they had abscesses when I was born? Once, in a quiet and intimate Rosen session, a sensitive practitioner touched the tiny remaining scars; I felt then for a second the searing pain of that long-ago surgery. I mentioned this when the surgeon asked if my breasts had ever been "traumatised". The lump, incidentally, is just at the end of the scar on the left nipple.

Or is there some still unknown trauma around the death of my beloved Big Granny, Grandmother Wyatt, who died a very painful death of breast cancer in the early 1940s? A picture of her in hospital floated up as I wrote that last sentence. Cancer treatment was in its early stages in those days; she was greatly deformed and in much pain. I never really understood her death; she just disappeared out of my life. There one day with her wonderful love and sense of fun, and gone the next. Ingrid and I worked through my panic and confusion as an eight-year-old, when such a beloved and integral part of my life just disappeared. This is where control, the lack of control over our lives surfaces. We think we are in control, then bang, cancer, death, illness, pain, panic and confusion. What control? Control is only an illusion of the mind it appears.

What else have I set up for myself? Fear I suppose — with me to the bitter end no doubt! Fear of the unknown, one of my most basic feelings, and here at every turn. Fear of the surgery, the treatment, the outcome, the future and, at its most basic, my ability to handle all this, to cope. You name it, I fear it! I recently read an allegedly helpful article in the Womens' Weekly concerning the courage of a well-known actor in handling his cancer of a gland in the neck. I didn't find it all that helpful to be told of his courage and triumph over adversity. I don't feel courageous at all, can only find courage within from time to time. Most times I am scared out of my wits and my stomach leaps and lurches all over the place, quite out of control.

Let's have all the cards on the table. Although the thought of tomorrow's surgery gives me the shivers — my poor left breast, as if it had not had enough to contend with. It is also the thought of the follow up treatment, should it be malignant, which gives me the creeps.

I speak of radiotherapy and, in particular, chemotherapy. The prospect of the former I find I can handle, just. OK the rays are harmful, deadly, but at least they will be bombarded only into a restricted area on my left side. The latter, having poison pumped throughout my whole system, so that I am nauseous and my hair falls out, just sends me freaking off again. In fact I sat in my sitting room in the early hours of the morning one night this week and considered the possibility I might even refuse to have it. Again I should add I am anticipating here. The lump may not be malignant; even if it is, chemotherapy may not be required if it is small and well contained. Pain, the Yogis say, is minimised by living in the present, neither looking back, nor forward. Just hanging in the present, one hour at a time, that's enough.[81]

I went to bed last night reasonably calm and peaceful. I awoke, some hours later, with my stomach all over the place. I grabbed my own scribble book — my journal — opened it at random, seeking

[81] See also *The Angel of Pain*, p. 292

something, anything to steady me. I found myself reading a piece I wrote in early 1993, my short giving birth, the rebirth of Judith, piece.[82] The imagery in that piece is powerful. It steadied me as I wrote it, it steadied me again as I re-read it this morning.

As I look back on the past eighteen months since we came to live in Tumut, much of my life both inner and outer has been of birth and re-birth: of letting go old patterns and slowly acquiring new feelings. As I read this morning it floated through my mind that perhaps my current situation was also one of healing and re-birth. I wonder if my childhood abuse (minor though it was) and the consequential denial of certain aspects of my feminine, could have been involved in the formation of this famous or infamous lump. I don't know. So this blockage has to be removed and the area treated; the healing.

The process of going through this healing is a process of rebirth, psychological and spiritual. See how the scenario sets up all the requisites. I am out of control, have to accept, am fearful of the unknown, doubting of my ability to cope and need practice in learning to trust.

See also the acceptance required at every turn: I need to be tender, loving, gentle with myself; not hassle myself for freaking, being so fearful, so panicky. It's a tough spot for anyone, take it quietly, one day at a time. It's all right to be upset, quite all right. Go gently with yourself, Judith, handle yourself lovingly, firmly as you would a frightened child. All will be well.

Gently, gently, gently...

---

82 See *"He came oh, so still…* p. 192

Heartache

Dear Friend,

Hello? Two letters in just a few days! That says something about my life at the moment. A lump in my breast — with the very real possibility of cancer — for which I had surgery a few days ago under a general anaesthetic. And now this last weekend, despite all the other upheaval, we have had the family party we planned some months ago to celebrate my sixtieth birthday and christen my beloved yurt. It has been an eventful two and a half weeks! I feel as if I have lived a lifetime since that fateful Thursday morning of the diagnosis.

Last week I wrote of being out of control, of the panic, the fear of the unknown involved in all of this, of having to accept, of the possibility that this was all part of a process of rebirth. Today other issues come to mind.

Despite the absence of the results of the pathology report, I start from my own near conviction that the lump will prove to be malignant. This puzzles me; I am normally logical, sensible and not given to pessimism; in fact on most matters I am optimistic. The research shows that genetically breast cancer is carried through the female line; yet it was my paternal grandmother who died of it. In cases such as mine, research also shows that nine out of ten lumps are benign. On both counts therefore the research gives me a good chance. Why am I so sure then that my lump is of the one in ten malignant variety?

An intuitive compassionate woman who works in a hospice in Melbourne came to visit just after my news broke. Talking quietly, we speculated that this might be an experience I needed to have: that, for whatever reason, irrespective of the results of the pathology, I needed to experience three weeks of dreading, fearing, expecting breast cancer. And, if I am honest, it is not just in the last three weeks. Breast cancer has been one of my secret fears or dreads for as long as I can remember

Let me ask myself the classic bodyworker's question: what is my body trying to tell me? Can I identify repressed feelings that might be involved in this tumour, or look for reflections in the mirror? Is my body trying to help by bringing forward insights into hidden parts of my personality? The tumour was a small lump on the left breast; in fact the lowest stich from the surgery is just above the nipple. It is that lowest stitch just above my heart that still aches and throbs from time to time. Writing that sentence I have gone all shivery inside, tears are coming; heartache, my heading. What is this about?

In bodywork terms, breasts in general are about sexuality, femininity, and nourishing. During my Rosen sessions with Ingrid I saw my breasts involved in all three areas. If nothing else, my feelings around my own sexuality would certainly now be involved in my fears of a mutilating mastectomy. If I look at the scar from my initial surgery, it is only about two inches long and quite neat. I find I can live with that which is an enormous relief.

In terms of femininity my Rosen work established that my encounter with Tom sent much of my own Aphrodite type femininity into hiding[83]. Now that I have rediscovered this late in life it seems to have taken on a treasure-like richness, a wonder, almost a magic, if you like, which may not have been present, if it had always been a part of my life. Hence the shivering, sobbing pain I felt at the thought that someone, anyone, but in particular a male surgeon, might slice into my breast with a scalpel. I simply could not face the thought that my now recovered treasured femininity might be wounded yet again.

Finally, there is the nourishing aspect. My sessions with Ingrid unearthed a deep and continuing grief at my inability as a mother to breastfeed my own children — caused by that long-ago surgery on the abscesses. I found there shame and deep feelings of inadequacy as a woman; a condemning of myself out of hand. Now as I look in the mirror I see more. There is still, many years later, a deep and abiding continuing grieving, a loss, a heartache; I am at loss for the appropriate word. It sounds mad, but it is true, I grieve and deeply, to this day that I

---

83 See *Through a Glass Darkly*, p. 116

could not breastfeed my own children. When my children left this morning, I noticed my stitches throbbed. Was my heart aching because this group of people dear to me was leaving? Is this where I have been all these years, broken hearted because I couldn't breastfeed my own young? This much seems undeniable; but there must be more to it than that.

Louise L. Hay in her booklet on the possible metaphysical causation for physical illness suggests that tumours may come into existence through the nursing of old hurts and shocks. More specifically under cancer, she lists deep hurt and deep grief eating away at the self, suggesting that remorse, resentment and depression are some of the repressed feelings involved.[84] I can't find these in myself at the moment, although a full Rosen session might unearth them. Yet I have only to touch the thought of failing to breastfeed my own children and the tears rise. Deep grief, all these years later.

If this is so, and it is certainly how I feel it at the moment, then this yearning to nourish my own young is a near obsession. Suddenly, as I write, I have glimpsed another perspective. Metaphorically bodywork, teaching, and writing, opening people's minds to ideas, to possibilities they may find valuable in their lives are all forms of nourishing. Maybe there are experiences here I need to have.

It can be easy for the life of any health care professional to become an ego trip: look how I help other people, look what a great person I am, is an easy enough trap. I have had cancer survivors as clients; I thought I knew something of what they were going through. I now know this was arrant nonsense; I had at best the merest inkling. I suspect I could have appeared, or even been, patronising about another's pain, in this one of the most feared of all painful diseases. I have been greatly humbled. Maybe all people who work with emotional pain at a very deep level, need to be where I have been.

Another revelation has been the intensity of my panic and fear of total disintegration under the weight of this pain. I found I couldn't handle sympathy or any spoken understanding at all. The thought of it

---

[84] Louise L. *Hay, Heal Your Body*, Specialist Publications, Sydney, 1986

terrified me; I feared it would push me right under. That too was a new experience for me and probably necessary.

Previously, as I now see it, I have raced into another's pain offering help, support, compassion, whatever. Never before, even when my mother died, have I not been able to accept the help and support of others. Again I have been humbled. I have seen some of my previous offers of help as possibly over enthusiastic, naive or immature at best, and as down right ego driven at worst.

Finally, to my surprise I have found myself ashamed to think I could have cancer. I found myself judging myself, condemning myself for having repressed grief, remorse, and resentment — feelings that in my view almost certainly contribute to malignant tumours. Yet when I have worked with cancer survivors, I have always put to them that all these feelings are deeply unconscious so that in no way can there be any question of responsibility, blame or guilt. Yet here I am condemning myself when, at least outwardly, I was not condemning others.

So it is beginning to appear that I have a near addiction to nourishing, helping others and a few problems that need attention along the way. Working with Ingrid, I learnt something of the handling of addictions: to recognise them for what they are, to accept them. Then gradually the addictive behaviour begins to wane. It seems that now is the time for me to appreciate the intensity of my need to help, to nourish others and to attempt to move beyond it. On the horizon now loom very real possibilities of nourishing in many ways: new grandchildren, clients, visitors to the yurt and readers of my book. But this nourishing must be sensitive and balanced.

This last weekend was such a happy one despite the odds. Was it a christening and a welcome to a new way of life? I think so; I trust so. I had invited our children, their partners, the grandchildren and some of my cousins — my "as if" siblings. Jill, Jim, Sam and their unborn second child occupied the yurt — new life[85]. They organised an afternoon tea of scones and jam and cream to formalise the christening. The yurt, let's remember is circular, without internal barriers, light, airy, stunning. I

[85] Jill, our eldest daughter, Jim her husband and "Sam" (Samantha our eldest granddaughter, then five). Jill and Jim were expecting another baby in about two months.

could write a book on its symbolism.

Together the whole group planted forty-nine of the eighty-five bushes for my rose hedge. This is a big imaginative project in which the boundary between the garden and the cattle is a part of the garden. Sceptics abound; the roses will neither be thick enough nor prickly enough to deter the cattle. My meditation and the literature say otherwise.

Thus we launched two fundamental Tumut projects with the help and blessing of my support group. The feelings I found from this weekend surprised me greatly. I expected exhaustion and tears — generally upset and confused feelings, for the outcome of the pathologist's report was still hanging over our heads. Not so. On that sunny Sunday morning as we laughed and planted, strength and a sense of quiet confidence came flooding in. I can't tell you how beautiful this was. To feel I could cope, would survive, had the inner strength and the confidence to take each day quietly as it came.

I have written previously of my old fear, with me to the bitter end. On one of my recent sleepless nights I was sitting musing on that phrase in front of the dying fire. Suddenly it struck me that I had the feelings for my fear one would have for an old and well known friend: a trusty companion, an integral part of every scene! My mind jumped sideways; I looked again. Now I seemed to have no fear of this fear and, lo, when that happens, suddenly, one can be serene. I have gone still as I write; my pen moves slowly. Ever since I was a teenager I have prayed for two things — wisdom and serenity. Wisdom, I have seen slowly coming my way these last few years; but serenity has always seemed beyond my grasp. Yet now, what is this I feel?

If I can allow myself to be out of control, quietly and trustingly accepting the situation, feeling strong and sufficiently confident to take each day gently as it comes, then I no longer need be afraid of being afraid. And then, Friend, joy of joys, I am serene. We shall see…

It's a few days later, now. We went to see the surgeon yesterday; I knew what he was going to say and I was not mistaken: that nasty little lump is a very early cancer. As we spoke I held in my mind an image of my beloved dancer: she was on centre stage, hands folded quietly, feet still, at rest, but poised ready to move[86]. I was able to take the news quietly without tears or fuss. We moved to a discussion of the next phase of treatment: more surgery and/or radiation therapy.

I have come a long way these last three weeks. I feel as if I have finally grown up. A curious feeling at sixty!

Who knows what tomorrow brings!

[86] See *The Dancer Within*, p. 144, *The Heart's Wisdom*, p. 195 and *Idling*, p. 182

The Inferno — A Nasty Experience

Suddenly, today the full import of my cancer has finally hit me. In a rage over some trivial detail, I heard myself shout, "I don't know, I have cancer, leave me alone". A few seconds later I realised that I had probably heard, really heard deep inside me, for the first time that phrase, "I have cancer". I saw then that I have used other phrases, "my lump is unfriendly", "it is malignant" (which is a meaningless phrase for me). Most often I talk of my "brush with cancer", a phrase I coined myself. This seems to enable me to talk of it to others and myself without upsetting any of us too much. One thing I learnt early on was that my news had the capacity to upset others. You have to be careful how you tell people you have cancer. You have also to be prepared for a staggering variety of responses.

Why does the word cancer stir so much? Is it because it can be terminal so that for many people it is their first brush with mortality? Is it the physical and emotional pain involved? Or is the fear of the unknown present here? The causes of cancer, unknown; the chances of recurrence, difficult to assess with certainty; the methods of treatment, various; their effects on individual bodies, varying. Yes, fear of the unknown is certainly a large part of it for me.

What is it that really upsets me? My own mortality, or mortality generally? Is it lurking there in the depths of my unconscious? It could be; but I would need a Rosen session to unearth that. Moreover, from day one, plans and projects for my own future have continued to eventuate. The yurt, my beloved yurt, is completed; surely I am to be around to develop that. Aspects of my book, my Rosen practice and my proposed garden continue to surface. I have to deal with them despite my current fuzzy state. It is impossible to believe I am about to die when surrounded by so much life and living. Quite simply, I don't believe it.

Now what of pain; I have written of my terror of a mastectomy and of chemotherapy. That is very nasty. For the mastectomy, it is not so much the physical pain that I fear, as the mutilation and the ensuing emotional and psychological trauma. In the case of chemotherapy, I have an absolute horror of what it would do to my body, and whether I would have the strength to survive. It's odd, isn't it; it is neither the vomiting nor the diarrhoea that terrify me so much as the hair loss.[87] Is it simply that for me the consequences of hair loss are unknown, whereas after many years of living in Asia, an upset stomach is an old friend? Or am I one of the Samson's of this world? Is my curly springy hair a source of strength? I must confess I have always found it so. I find it hard to be my usual vibrant self when my hair goes straight and flat, after childbirth or surgery.

What else remains of pain? Last week I had an appointment at the Wagga Wagga Base Hospital with a visiting oncologist from Sydney, said by my Tumut surgeon to be an expert in his field. We were to seek his advice as to the further course of treatment — further surgery and radiation therapy or radiation only. Neither Ian nor I had realised the implication of being amidst the clamour and chaos of a cancer clinic at a big public hospital.

We arrived to a small dark room on the south side of the building with people milling everywhere. There were some nice touches: a welcoming cup of coffee for country patients; a volunteer "cancer survivor" who made it his business to talk quietly to new patients of the various services provided. Beyond that, the room was crowded with patients in varying

---

[87] Chemotherapy drugs have improved greatly in the ten years since this was written. Vomiting and diarrhoea are much less frequent and more easily controlled. "Spare the hair" drugs can now be used in some cases.

stages of cancer awaiting either chemotherapy or a session with the doctor. Here we waited two hours as the clinic was "running late"!

Ian found it difficult: he was irritated by the inefficiency of the delay and that we were never warned of it. We could have gone for a walk sparing ourselves a little. I was simply traumatised by the pain and suffering in the room: there were two women minus a breast, a man and a woman who could barely make themselves understood (cancer of the larynx). There were others with faces and body language dark with pain, suffering and despair. Most did not look as if they really understood what was going on. They sat despairingly, ignorantly and powerlessly waiting. Dear God it was awful; I can't describe just how awful it was. Waiting in that clinic, it came to me that living through serious forms of cancer is a twentieth century version of hell. Who needs visions of an afterworld replete with suffering and damnation, when cancer of the larynx will provide it here and now? The Inferno…

Finally, my turn came, not yet with the great man himself, but with a young specialist in training. He took my medical history, gave me a quick examination and then his advice: to take off the whole breast and all associated lymph nodes was the only way to ensure no stray cancer cell remained. I hung onto myself literally — arms crossed shielding both breasts — pulled myself, my intelligence, my education, my training together and set out to protect my body. I seem to tread a fine line at the moment. I don't want to die of cancer, yet on the other hand, both my training and intuition say "minimal surgery": a body is designed to function as a whole, no one piece should be removed, therefore, unless it is absolutely essential. So I replied as firmly as I could manage that I didn't want the surgery unless it was absolutely imperative and what were the other alternatives.

In due course I saw the great man himself, older, quieter and wiser. His view was that in ten years time more surgery and radiation would almost certainly give the same results as radiation alone. In those circumstances my intuition and training won out, there would be no further surgery.

Later as we lunched in Wagga, I was just barely hanging on to myself:

hysterics (which I have never had) would have been easy. I had this dreadful feeling I could just fall apart, disintegrate under the strain. It stayed all through the hour-long car trip home. On a quiet stroll up the hill to see the first lambs, twins as it happened, tears poured down my face.

What is it about that morning that affected me so very strongly? The hairs on my head are tingling as I write. I can't stop thinking about it, talking about it. What is this about? When I started this piece I thought I had simply been deeply affected by the pain of others; this now seems unlikely. One doesn't have this depth or strength of reaction confronted by another's pain. So the scene is triggering something in me, in my own unconscious. Put another way, it hooks into and pulls to the surface my own pain. So what was so diabolically painful for me in that cancer clinic?

A few days later I had a Reiki session with a friend. My trip to Wagga surfaced again. This time I saw my own place in the scene. By the Grace of God I was youngish (many of the others would have been seventy plus), sufficiently educated to have some glimpse of an understanding of what was going on, privately insured, with enough assets to have the best possible care and supported by a loving husband. Last, but by no means least, my cancer was minimal. This time I am blessed, no doubt about that. If I have to have cancer for some reason, I am in the best possible situation to deal with it.

And the others? Is this where the inferno, my version of hell comes in? Old, very old some of them, not necessarily understanding what had happened to them, what now had to be done, and trapped in the relative anonymity of the public health system. So there they sit silently, patiently, powerlessly, suffering. The suffering, the pain caused by ignorance and powerlessness is mind blowing. I feel it as I write: my stomach is beginning to flutter, my writing has slowed right down. I can feel how deeply moved I am at this point: the suffering of ignorance, the pain of it, my inferno...

Here I find myself again — obsessed, drugged, whatever word you want to use. I have to understand, will flay myself, my friends, colleagues, teachers, anyone, even my enemies in order to find out. I am driven by a compulsive craving to understand what is happening and why. If I look back, this need has driven the development of the whole course of my life: my love of books, of research, of learning, of scholarship, my curiosity about people, how they live their lives, about governments, institutions and all things. My favourite story in Kipling's *Just So Stories*, is the *Elephant's Child*, with his "satiable curiosity". Curiosity carried me through many a mundane diplomatic event. I blessed it every time. I am rarely bored. I can always wonder why something should be so and float away.

So, for me to sit ignorant, despairing, suffering would be my own private form of hell. No wonder the scene in that Wagga clinic grabbed me and held me so hard. No wonder I felt that I might fall apart.[88] My inferno…[89]

[88] See also *Judith Ann Wyatt (Nicholson)*, p. 235 for further insights into my feelings at that cancer clinic.

[89] See p. 216

O Ye of Little Faith

I just seem to have feelings powering out of me at the moment. It all seems relevant, and I fear I may forget some. Oh ye of little faith! Yes, ye of little faith, that describes me just now. And those of us with little faith struggle and struggle to control our lives for fear of the unknown. Ah me, there have been tough lessons about this lately... Such is life.

Prior to my first appointment at the radiation oncology clinic at the Canberra Hospital, I had a confrontation with my fear of the unknown such as I have never had before. I went to bed with my bladder and groin aching and my very flesh crawling with this fear. "Fear of what?" asked Ian as he tried to comfort me. "I don't know," I had to reply, "yet I am so terrified, I seem to be immobilised, paralysed with this fear." Of all the words I have ever used, ever read, describing such a confrontation none now seemed adequate. Yet I must be able to find a metaphor. Previously, when precise words have failed I have said "it is as if..." Now, it is as if what? Ah, I have just seen the very nub of it. If I could describe the sensation of this fear, see an image of it, I would have named it, brought it in from the unknown mass, made it familiar in some way and thus eased my terror of the unknown.

As I spoke to Ian, I recalled a paragraph in Elaine Mayland's book on the Rosen Method describing an area of the body low in the torso where the legs and pelvis connect as that in which the deepest feelings of fear are often held. "This sort of fear," she writes, "seems to threaten one's very existence, one's very being, and is very deeply and tightly held. When that fear lets go, the struggle is gone from one's life, and the possibility of moving freely with life instead of holding against it becomes available."[90] Physically this made sense, for it was deep in my torso I was feeling this aching pain. So I grabbed a spare pillow, held it tightly against myself and finally fell asleep.

What is it about radiation that triggers this fear, seems to threaten my very existence? Ian said to me reasonably and sensibly, "Radiation has few side effects, why do you fear it so much?" To which I mutter sarcastically in reply, "Oh yes, only a few side effects, it can kill you if it's incorrectly used!" This, though, is to focus only on the physical. Yet the intensity of my feelings suggests my unconscious must be involved in some way, that it is to the psychological rather than the physical that I should look.

The words I find so gripping in Mayland's writing are those referring to the threat to one's existence, one's being. Most of the Yogi and other spiritual books I have read talk of ego loss, loss of feelings of the importance of self, as being one important aim of a spiritual journey. One merges into, dissolves, melts into God, the Self, the Divine, however you like to express it. The idea being that "I" have no aims or objectives other than those which the Divine has for me — acceptance in the proverbial nutshell. Certain it is that most egos freak at the loss of apparent control and importance involved in this proposition. They want to regard themselves as stars, on centre stage for every act in the drama of their particular life, whether as hero, heroine, villain or victim.

The question of the role of the ego in my spiritual life has puzzled me for years. Over time I have come to accept the writings of a medium called Bartholemew who suggests that egos are not so much lost as transformed.[91] If I expand this a little, I could say that if we postulate non-duality — that every single thing is part of the One — then it follows that my ego must also be Divine, be part of that One. If this is so, then on my

[90] See Elaine L. Mayland, *Rosen Method: An Approach to Wholeness and Well-being through the Body*, privately published, 8th Edition, 1996.

[91] Joy Franklin and Mary-Margaret Moore (eds) *Bartholomew, Reflections of an Elder Brother*, High Mesa Press, New Mexico, 3rd printing 1990, p. 139-140.

inner travels I and my ego are not going to fall apart in some excruciatingly terrifying unknown way, "we" are simply going to be even more than usually myself; very likely in a way unknown to my present conscious self but known to my unconscious. Years ago my meditation said I was to be a "grass roots" or "market place" mystic: there was to be no nunnery for me and no great dramatic declaration; I was simply to live my life like everyone else. In so doing I am the literal manifestation that every one of us is Divine just exactly as we are. All that is required is an awareness, an openness to that possibility.

So why am I to go to the radiation clinic? For healing of this current cancer, for protection against future cancers, for a transformation, a chance to live the rest of my life free from the unconscious canker, whatever it may be, that has been secretly eating into me from within all these years.

And the means of achieving this? I am to have tiny highly regulated doses of an awesome power, a healing power, directed to the exact spot. This reminds me of the comfort Amy has been offering these last few weeks: "Dearest Judith," she has been quietly insisting, "if everything is part of the One, part of the Divine, then so too is radiation. It cannot be only destructive as you see it, but must also offer healing." All I have to do is relax, try not to fear, not to obstruct the healing and just let it all happen. Be of good faith, in a word… I shall be trying hard to be relaxed and trusting. It may not be the easiest thing I have ever had to do.

Shadows on the Path

At long last I have come to Canberra for the radiation therapy. There have been days in the last three to four weeks — waiting for an appointment to have my radiation needs assessed, waiting for a slot to become available in the radiation program — when I thought this segment of my treatment would never begin. Frustration has been the name of the game: frustration by forces beyond my control and, as importantly, the ways in which I now understand I frustrate myself. Frustration by the "nasties" of this world, frustrating myself, I seem to be buried, inextricably entangled in frustration at the moment…

Recently Ian and I watched a segment on breast cancer on TV. I suppose people take from any program those things they are unconsciously seeking. Ian took a message of hope. To him it seemed we were being steered along the lines of the most highly regarded current form of treatment. He was therefore unprepared to come to bed after me, and find me sobbing as if my heart would break.

For my part, in watching the program, my unconscious had been hooked by the references to the many people who have multiple breast cancers. I saw the possibility of a future, in which although my life might be intact, I would spend all my time and energy, battling one cancer after another. Currently I detest the stories some of my would-be-helpful but rather insensitive friends tell of someone they know, who has had two mastectomies and chemotherapy, but is "absolutely fine now". My heart all but stops at the thought of the terror, the courage, the pain and suffering required to live through all that, in order to be "absolutely fine now".

What came to me after that TV program was an almost overwhelming grief. I had spent thirty-five years of my adult life being wife of Ian, mother to our four children, daughter and daughter-in-law. Ian and I had agreed that on his retirement and our move to Tumut, I was going to have my chance to live *my* life and do *my* thing. It had looked, until a few weeks ago, as if it was all falling beautifully into place. Man had proposed, surely God was not now going to dispose by setting me up to spend the rest of my life battling cancer in one form or another. I thought my heart would break.

Tears are pouring down my face as I write, am I never to have my chance? I seem to have something to offer; am I to go quietly to my grave with it all still locked inside? Is this just an ego trip? It certainly looks that way. It doesn't feel like that to me; it feels like an aching need for fulfilment; as if there is a great empty void within crying to be made whole by the use of the gifts I now know I have. It was a nasty, nasty night.

In a remote intellectual way I could see that this grief could be lessened by trust. If I could just trust that cancer was an experience I needed to have; trust that all my other projects would also develop; then clearly I could still be serene. On that particular night trust was as far away as Mars; there was no way of drawing anywhere near it. I have just realised though that framed that way I am still on an ego trip. For I am trusting that my ego needs will be met!

I realised when I received the cancer diagnosis that a fundamental part of this experience would be that of being out of control, almost totally without power. Within some limits, doctors would treat me how, where and when they deemed appropriate. I would be expected to flow gracefully and gratefully on. For let us remember, medical science is offering me back my life. I thought I was prepared for that, I knew it was inevitable. What I didn't realise at the time, was that in setting up a proposed trip to the United States of America once the cancer treatment was finished, I was by implication trying to control the timing of the treatment itself. It was a grim lesson to learn.

Mark lives in Washington.[92] By a strange coincidence, on the day I had planned to ring him to tell him of the cancer diagnosis, he rang to ask me to visit him and meet my newest grandchild due in two or three weeks time. Given the vagaries of the cancer treatment, we agreed that I would go as soon as I could, preferably in early November, since he would in any event be coming to Australia with his family for Christmas. He offered to pay part of my fare. I was really touched and excited, it seemed like a wonderful break, a chance to put a space between me and my cancer. "Full stop, new paragraph," was how I described this trip to myself.

Then there was a phone call from the radiation clinic: one of the machines had broken down, my commencement date would have to be delayed again, throwing doubts on my proposed trip to the United States. It was beginning to appear pointless; I would no sooner arrive than they would be preparing to leave for Australia. Curious, isn't it how one very small change can break down a dam of repressed feelings. Frustration entered the scene again. Was every aspect of my life to be entangled in this cancer round forever?

In bed that night, I found myself caught up in an emotional storm the intensity of which I have never experienced before. It was not grief this time, but rage, fury, a blinding white searing anguish, that I could be caught, inexorably, in such a trap. No way to avoid cancer, no way to avoid the treatment with its timing foibles. This is life, it has to be accepted.

I sobbed, shivered, thumped the bed, roared and ranted like a mad thing. It was no use. There seemed to be something deeper, some basic block at the very depth of my being. As Ian gently rubbed my back, I began to cough, I thought I would vomit. And then came a picture of myself held as if in a vice by iron bars, trapped and caged. I heard myself howl the howl of an animal trapped, suffering, maddened beyond endurance. I had once heard a fellow student make a similar noise in an

---

92 Mark our only son and second child, was at that time working for the World Bank and living in Washington with his wife Alice.

early Rosen training session. I watched practitioner and student continue quietly; I marvelled at their courage, for that howl had gone through me like a knife. I had not known such emotional agony existed.

Now I had made that same noise myself. My ego, face to face with the inexorable and unflinching demands of the Divine, had finally howled itself out. I lay spent, shivering in the bed. I turned to Ian: "I am sorry," I said, "I imagine you were as frightened as I was when I first heard that noise. It's O.K., though, I am all right now." So he went off to sleep, and I went to the kitchen for the inevitable cup of tea. And then, yes, I slept too, of exhaustion no less.

There's the first strand, then, total, absolute, utter frustration at the inexorable demands of the Divine. I know of no words to convey what I felt that night. It was as if every fibre of my being was howling at my inability to be able to do what I wanted. And this has to be ego stuff, pure and simple. Dear God this is what I want from my life, please. Answer — No — Grrrh…

However, the delay in the radiation clinic brought up another aspect of frustration: those situations where, in effect, I frustrate myself. When Ian and I talked of the possible delay the following morning, I was really upset. Ian was comforting and consoling. We have different memories of our actual conversation. It seemed to me that he was saying in a very nice way that my departure date in November was becoming so late that it was a bit silly (for which I read extravagant and not sensible) to be considering the trip at all, for Mark would soon be here. In other words I thought he thought I shouldn't go. In which case note, I, Judith, in all probability won't go, no matter how much I want to. Now there are two separate elements here. He denies he put it that way; in which case I am projecting. But irrespective of what he said, I know I will deny myself something I want to do because of the views of another. At this point I am frustrating myself.

Later that morning I rang Amy for comfort. She asked a few illuminating questions among which was a bull's eye: "Forgive me asking," she said in her lovely English voice, "but don't you have money of your own?

Can't you spend that on yourself, on any project you yourself want to undertake?" "We don't treat our money separately in that way," I replied, "and, if I spent it on something of which Ian disapproved, I would feel guilty." "Guilt," she murmured, "yes, of course, I understand."

As I put the receiver down a whole chunk of my inner life was suddenly illuminated. I appear on the surface, to go after what I want. In truth though, I manoeuvre endlessly trying to ensure that everyone else wants what I want. If it appears there can be no agreement, then either I do what every one else wants (be this fear of rejection, the good girl, or a desire for harmony) or I go my own way, but feeling guilty. The minutiae of psychoanalysis are irrelevant. What I saw with such blinding clarity that morning was how very seldom I actually decide what I want to do and then do it, simply, clearly and untrammelled by a myriad of negative emotions. The circumstances were frustrating me, yes, but they were also illustrating the extent to which I frustrate myself. All my unconscious baggage was constantly muddying the waters.

Once Amy's questions had illuminated the problem, it was easily solved. A few family conversations showed that Ian was in fact quite relaxed about timing, but that Mark and I for different reasons both wanted a visit as soon as the radiation permitted. Clarity at last. I took the decision that I would go in November. Ironically, on arrival in the clinic on Monday morning, I was told the situation had changed again; I should finish earlier than feared, thus few problems with the November date!

This has become very long yet the depth and intensity of the feelings seems to suggest that it is very important in some way. Let's see if I can pull it all together. Writing of my aching need for fulfilment, I said I hoped it was not ego stuff. "Yes, I can see it now; I was deluding myself; it was ego stuff pure and simple. Why should I expect to lead what I regard as a fulfilled life? The Divine does not owe me the life I want. That is, it must be ego stuff."

So how does it work then? I have spent much time this last week meditating, snoozing on my bed. It has come to me that each one of us is given the gift of a life, a gift from the Divine and together with each life come the gifts required to use that particular life to fulfil the Divine purpose.

If this is so, then I am where I am supposed to be and have the necessary gifts to do whatever it is that I am supposed to do. Then I can choose either to set my own goals and struggle endlessly frustrated if they do not coincide with those of the Divine; or I can try to ascertain and flow with the Divine pattern, making use of the Divine gifts. Either way, I have the required gifts and can be fulfilled, so long as I let my own goals fade. A life without frustration, a dream, I wonder...

There seems, also, to be one very important final point: whatever I choose to do I have to be clear and true, to who and what I am, what I believe in, what I need for myself from others, as well as what others need for themselves from me. We are each as important as the next guy, not more so, not less so. Unless this is very clear the waters all around us are constantly muddied as we do what we think we should, ought or must do. We need to recognise that we don't understand the whole plan. We shouldn't try to. We have to be still and clear each of us in our own spot.

Recently I was given a CD of Artur Rubenstein playing Chopin waltzes — wondrous music — such purity and clarity in every note. Each mote has its own value and each is heard in its appointed place in exquisite harmony. This must be how life can be if we are each true to ourselves and our place in the Divine music. I have finally finished week one of my radiation therapy. What a long way I have come! For the moment I feel calm, serene, at peace.

On Being Squeezed

I *am about half way through my six weeks of radiation* and in a really bad way. Since I have a severe attack of radiation shakes and trembles, I am supposed to be resting quietly on my bed; that only seems to make it worse. So I have resorted to a loved and trusted option — steadying myself with the written word. I have being doing this for years now; to date it has never failed. So here goes.

It was in Tumut recently over a weekend, that I began to have insights into a very different form of lovemaking. Aspects of this, words, feelings, murmurings came drifting in on the wind, as it were. It was all quite exquisitely beautiful, almost beyond words.

The basic proposition seemed to be that one moved into making love not so much from feelings of lust or desire to enjoy the body of one's partner; nor from any feelings of wanting to have one's own body similarly stirred. Rather, as I felt it, each partner had the vision, the yearning, for a deeper experience, a union, which went way beyond the gratification of the desires of any individual body. In order that this union and the feelings involved in it might come about each partner trustingly offers up his/her body. The operative words are "offer up". One offers up one's body in order that the experience of this union may be made manifest. For me it was powerful — to offer up one's body.

Then my mind leapt sidewards. This must be what the cancer was requiring of me; that I offer up my body, in this case for healing, the transformation required. And as in sexual union so too in the cancer treatment, this has to be done trustingly, lovingly. If I pause here, this is in line with the whole of my spiritual journey. I have not been only on some odyssey of the intellect exploring philosophy and creeds. I have been, am, involved at every level of my being, intellect, feelings and, equally importantly, my body. My body has to be involved; trustingly put forward to allow what would manifest, to be manifested. And it comes to me as I write, that to put one's body forward is the hardest part of all. One can change one's mind, alter one's feelings, yet once one's body is committed the situation is irreversible.

The following week on my return to Canberra I felt squeezed on every side. I had been most generously lent a house in Canberra by a close friend who is currently overseas. On my return from Tumut I found a mix-up in which relations of a girlfriend of one of my "landlord's" sons were indefinitely occupying what I had thought was my bed and without my permission. Since I was single they had moved my things out of the double bedroom I had previously been using and I was now occupying a single bedroom, used largely as a storeroom. I found myself sleeping surrounded by crates, boxes and posters of Exterminator II. I was not amused.

On the Tumut front, all our three daughters announced separately that they would come home the following weekend, each bringing a partner, friend, and in one case grandchildren. As you know we are a very happy and united family and my cancer has been a real blow to all of us. In theory such a weekend could be a special family time for us to be together and support each other. In practice, though, the weekend loomed as a continuation of the squeezing and lack of physical and psychological space I was feeling in Canberra. Since I could feel my anger rising and hear a frantic obsessive tone in my voice that warned me my unconscious was involved in some way, I sought the help of Irja, the social worker attached to the oncology unit at the hospital.

It is wonderful how easy it becomes to deal with unconscious material when someone objective helps from outside. Irja asked the most obvious, the most sensible question. "How do you see your cancer?" Immediately the image was there: a great black/green evil grasping thing, spreading its tentacles throughout every part of my body, and squeezing, squeezing, squeezing me until I had no room to move, could scarcely breathe. Suddenly everything fell into place. I was feeling squeezed to death by the cancer. Little wonder then, I felt so intensely all this physical and psychological squeezing.

And, in a very obvious, literal, physical sense I am being squeezed by the cancer at the moment. I can't live at home, can't wear a bra, can't wear most of my nice clothes because of the burn dressings, have to go daily to the hospital, have to survive the mood swings, the surfacing emotions, have to put just about all of my energies into living through cancer. I have no time, no energy for the outside world. I feel totally self — centred, self — absorbed. I hate to feel like this. But I have no energy left, no concentration span for anything else. I could feel my rage as I spoke of some of this. One phrase kept pounding through my mind: "out of my way, I want to get on with my life".

Irja suggested that I visualise the cancer out of me, which we hope it is, since the tumour itself has been excised. What would I do with it, she wanted to know, if I found it lying on the path in front of me or lying on the beach. If it were on the beach, I said, I would chop it into the most minuscule pieces and throw them into the sea; if on the path I would simply step over it and sweep on.

I was not confident of either of these reactions, although the feeling of assertion as I stepped over and swept on felt good. This was clearly the feeling she was hoping to attract — one in which I was on top of the cancer and it was no longer on top of me. Yet I kept remembering both Amy and Ingrid stressing that feelings had to be integrated not rejected. I don't intend to pursue that further here. It did feel good to have asserted myself vis-à-vis the cancer, and I now felt able to face the girls happily for the weekend. In the short term that was all I wanted.

In later insights I saw this squeezing connected with my deeply felt fear of a secondary cancer. We have not talked of this. Clinically mine was a small tumour in the earliest stage of development. Treated with surgery, radiation and possibly drugs for a couple of years no one stray cell should regrow in other parts of my body. There is thus supposed to be little danger of secondary cancer for me. And yet, and yet... in the dead of night I have this same nasty picture of a black evil being spreading deep in my very being and destroying me. When someone talks of secondary cancers, I feel my abdomen tighten and quiver. And, of course, at the hospital I am constantly exposed to those with secondary cancer. Those who are free from it are out in the community living their lives.

At some point my mind jumped from the physical/emotional to the spiritual/psychological. Then I began to see that squeezing experience at other levels of my being. As I have written over the weeks, one very large part of my cancer experience has to do with acceptance and with the loss, or transformation of my ego. My body and I are being put through the mill, as it were. My ego has to learn that it is no longer in control, does not call the shots, has to accept — and gracefully — that events may happen it would not seek, does not like. No wonder I have felt very confused recently. These are tough experiences, very tough indeed.

Somehow or other, I have to find trust. I have to learn to live the rest of my life "in remission", trusting that there will be no secondary cancer. When we moved to Tumut I wrote of trust and my struggle to learn to trust my meditation/intuition. In a sense, though, that was trust of a lesser kind. If our venture proved unsuccessful we could have pulled out at any time subject to possible financial and domestic upheavals. With cancer though, it is different. I have to trust, have to accept, there can be no pulling out; there is no alternative.

So my ego has taken a fearful battering these last few months and has reacted, I suppose, with the intense emotional storms I have been experiencing. Although I have written of one only of these, there have been three or four. I am easily moved and cry often. These storms, though, are something again: there is a depth of feeling, an intensity of feeling that shakes me to my core. I feel as though I am being torn, ripped apart. Ian holds me, rocks me as you would a distraught child; we are both, I think, not a little frightened at their severity. Is this the reaction of the ego as it feels itself uprooted from its previously perceived position of dominance, pre-eminence? It could be.

Judith Ann Wyatt (Nicholson)

Dear Friend,

I seem to have been writing bits of this piece in my head for days now, hesitating to put pen to paper. The reason? Quite easy really. I want to keep it simple, and I want to have it "right" whatever that may mean.

For whom, I wonder, does it have to be right? After all, it's my story and in one sense I can tell it any way I like. It can even be pure fantasy. That's what scientists say when I tell them I work with my unconscious. "Oh that," they answer, in varying degrees of politeness and scepticism. "Oh, you can't prove that." And, of course, I can't, that's true. Yet when I am receiving a Rosen Session and my body gives an involuntary sigh, as if to say, "yes, that's it, that's what this is all about", that reaction brings it's own undeniable stamp of truth. Scientists may talk about objective proof, In unconscious matters I have the proof that matters to me — it feels right.

So, what am I on about that I need to be so firm and explicit that only my view is relevant? In a nutshell, my view of myself, which may be different from views of me held by others. What does it feel like to be Judith Wyatt, yes, my maiden name, one I haven't thought of for decades? In this context, though, that name feels right, for the basic personality traits of Judith, as she now is, were established long before she married, when she was Judith Wyatt.

Let's pause on the thorny subject of names. There is something quite kinky here. I find on reflection that I hardly have a name by which others call me to which I relate. Despite my advancing years and my slight embarrassment, my mother called me "Babe" till she died when I was fifty-six. My father called me "Duck", always, never anything else;

I loved that, still do. I had no brothers and sisters to invent pet names. School friends, colleagues, associates, friends of my adult life, call me Judith — a name to which I don't relate very well. Only if someone calls me Judy do I respond, and in anger. For, if I don't feel as if I am Judith, I do know I am not Judy; my father had very strong views on that! Ian for some reason known only to himself sometimes calls me "Hook".

Only two of the many names I go by seem to carry much meaning for me. A small group calls me "Mrs Nick"; I like that. It is a name to which I can relate, I know and understand Mrs Nick. When names for grandmothers were being discussed, I knew I did not want to be Granny or Nanna. I selected the name "Abba" for myself although I had no knowledge of its derivation. I don't know too much about Abba yet, maybe my growing band of grandchildren will teach me! What have I set up for myself, though, Friend? It is beginning to appear as if I may have an identity problem, as if perhaps I don't know who or what I am. It seems as if I may be a chameleon simply responding howsoever others choose to call me and possibly being whatever they want me to be.

What is this about? Since these thoughts are coming to me when I am being treated for breast cancer, are they involved with it? Let's start with the physical. I speculated earlier that my cancer was almost certainly connected with my deep grief at my inability to breast feed my own young, and my growing awareness of my near addiction to the nourishing of others.[93] Now I can see that in those early days of my cancer saga I was using the mirror of life to look outward. Recently I have had much insistent pain in my left nipple, not from childhood surgery this time, but from the heat of the radiation. It was almost as if my body, through that pain, was trying to talk to me: "Come on, woman, for God's sake," it seemed to be saying, "have another look, can't you. How much more pain do you need in order to understand the deepest meaning of this cancer?" My burns from the radiation have been nasty.

So sitting quietly on a park bench one lovely spring afternoon, Jennifer and I went back together through those major traumas of my

---

[93] See *Heartache*, p. 210

childhood which involved breasts and nipples, trying to find some previously overlooked unconscious pattern. Nipples had been clearly involved in the nipple lancing at my birth. Since small children have a close association between mothers, breasts and nipples, we speculated that my confusion and distress around my mother's absence when Tony was born, were involved in some as yet unknown way. Then there was confusion and hazy feelings around sexuality at Point Leo, and my early sexual encounter with Tom in the sleep-out.

"Don't try to make links between these incidents with your conscious mind," Jennifer warned. "Sit quietly, revisit the imagery of each one and see what feelings come up for you." So nearly sixty years later, I let the imagery from those scenes flow through my mind again. Slowly, and to my surprise, I began to feel how strongly I had been affected by the noise, the rough-handling and confusion in each of those scenes, and the extent to which I was craving support and a return to the rhythmn of my own peaceful life. I could feel panic rising. Where was the quiet loving world to which I was accustomed with all the well-known support of loving cherishing parents? "Look," she said, "we missed that one, breast feeding is not only about physical nourishing but also loving support." Was this what the continuing pain in my left nipple was about? Did I need to look at my unconscious need for a life of quiet loving harmony and support, and realise how that need was affecting my adult psyche?

I think I probably come across as someone who goes after what she wants. Probably I alone really know to what lengths I will go to ensure harmony, particularly within my family. I actually feel almost panicky if a family storm threatens. University Law Faculty fracas used to affect me the same way. When my integrity drives me to act in a way that is not acceptable to my peers, bringing fears of disharmony, my stomach flutters and I feel as though I am walking on quicksand.

After I had talked to Jennifer that week, I had dinner with a close Faculty friend. In due course my experiences at the Wagga oncology clinic surfaced. Retelling my story to her husband, I was dismayed to hear the frantic timbre in my voice that always signals the presence of the unconscious. I had thought I had worked that out of my system when I wrote about the Inferno: the Judith who can't stand the powerless suffering that comes from ignorance, the Judith who is driven by a need to understand. Apparently not.[94] When we spoke a couple of days later, I apologised for my behaviour at dinner. I had been "over the top". "Not at all," she replied, "I recognised and respected the anger."

The word anger brought me up short. Although I had seen myself as panicky and close to hysteria in the clinic, I hadn't felt the anger. Now, though, I could feel my anger rising; and I was not only angry, I was simply furious and my poor left nipple was still throbbing. So look again, what unconscious pattern connects the nipple lancing, other experiences around breasts and the Wagga cancer clinic?

Suddenly I felt other feelings of powerless victims, trapped in inescapable situations, feelings I had missed when I first wrote of the Wagga cancer clinic. Victims, I saw in a flash, could be not only panicky and hysterical, but also downright furious and, yes, resentful. There is simultaneously, "how dare you!" and, "why is this happening to me?" I recalled then that when the nipple lancing first surfaced in a Rosen session in Sweden, the practitioner suggested I might be feeling anger. I didn't, perhaps couldn't, touch it then. Now, though, it was different. I could feel the anger and it was zipping through me.

Later that same week I took my growing anger to Irja. Anger was not a feeling to which I was accustomed, I said, not like my old friend fear! But now that it had been stirred by recent conversations, I seemed to be angry a great deal. I could be angry with almost anyone about anything. I was most uncomfortable with it.

Irja talked, then, of the healing "energy" which a body releases during life threatening situations and diseases. "It may feel like anger to you," she said, "for you say you have not really experienced the subtle range of feelings around assertiveness. In reality, though, what you are most likely feeling, is a flow of power that is enabling you to assert yourself in situations where previously you would possibly not have

---

94 See *The Inferno*, p. 216

done so. This happens in order to enable you to protect your body and your psyche. It is in effect the "fight" response from the phrase "fight or flight". My body gave one of its quiet involuntary sighs. What she was saying felt so right; it must be true for me.

As a tiny baby I had been powerless, unable to assert myself: had had to accept and suffer, enduring the nipple lancing and whatever came my way. Similarly my mother's absence, the events at Point Leo and in the sleep-out had simply to be endured. And, I have seen as I write, my harmony loving soul would rather endure without fuss, for fear of creating a storm. However, finally in that Wagga cancer clinic, my sixty-year-old self was goaded almost beyond endurance by the waiting and the surrounding pain. Finally brought to my feet as it were, to protect my own body and possibly my life, I rallied, asserted myself, and risking the displeasure of the doctor, rejected that first advice for a mastectomy.

This has become complicated, Friend, hasn't it? Something, though, tells me it is vitally important for me. How can I make it clear? Let's start with that scene in the Wagga cancer clinic, it seems to be fundamental. At first as I look at my fellow-sufferers, all I see is the extent to which I have always been driven to avoid the suffering and powerlessness that comes from ignorance. However, over the ensuing weeks two more repressed feelings — my need for loving support and harmony, and my growing anger — surface in circumstances such that they need to be fitted into the picture.

Now where does this leave me? No matter how others see me, I see myself as always dancing, manoeuvring, circling, trying to ascertain what others wish and then to achieve that at all costs — the harmony craving Judith. If, on occasion, we do what I want and others don't, I am still a loser, for then, I feel uneasy, anxious and guilty! It appears I am in a no win situation. I am either in self-denial or guilty.

We might now come back to the first issue I raised, that of name and possibly, identity. I don't seem to have a name to which I relate comfortably. I don't really seem to know what I want, what I stand for. I do and I don't! I am like a leopard endlessly changing my spots.

If you look at that whole picture, you might not be surprised to find me, this woman with cancer. I seem to have a life threatening emotional/psychological disease, an overwhelming desire for loving support and quiet harmony combined with the inability to know when and how to assert and protect myself and what I stand for. I have had in fact, a canker, something secret, insidious, gnawing away at me and making it impossible for me to make whatever is *my* unique contribution to this world. It is also, perhaps, not surprising that I have cancer in my breast. I am, so it appears, also quite unable to "nourish" myself by allowing myself to flow untrammelled along the lines suggested for me by my life.

We have come a long way in the past fourteen weeks. I, for one, am absolutely exhausted by the journey. The medical profession nearly kills you when it treats you for cancer. However, even as I write I know I could rally myself, find my power and lash out at any one who threatened me! Aha, I have changed for good, it seems.

Nearly done now, only two more zapping days (radiation sessions). Friday I leave the hospital and return to Tumut. It seems very fitting that this weekend brings the first group of guests to the Yurt: a group of five friends from Canberra who go away to explore life together every three or four months. The beginning of life after cancer. I do hope so.

Next week I go travelling, off to the United States of America and the United Kingdom, primarily to meet my newest grandson — Alasdair Wyatt Hill Nicholson and be with his proud parents. This trip is my good behaviour award, a chance to go somewhere new, start life again, a full stop, new paragraph, life after cancer trip.

Tamoxifem

Dear Friend,

Greetings from the depth of the Goobra on a cold, dank autumn day: no sun, no rain, no wind, just a cold that seeps into my bones, no amount of thick clothing, warm fires or hot drinks seems to help. Over the years I survived with relative ease the rigours of the tropics in Phnom Penh and the cold in Northern Sweden. Not this time.

The oncologist mentioned recently that feeling the cold was a possible after affect of radiation. I wonder. It seems more than just physical; I feel cold to the very marrow of my bones. It sounds fanciful, I know, but I feel as if my very soul is cold, and a picture of that scene in the sleep-out with Tom, what I regard as one of my out-in-the-cold images, keeps popping into my mind. What is this about?

My life has been uncertain and confused these last six months as I have struggled to regain some semblance of normality after my brush with breast cancer. A part of this has hinged around a possible third phase of treatment — the taking of Tamoxifem, an oestrogen-reducing drug. Since oestrogen facilitates growth for some varieties of breast cancer cells, it is sometimes thought prudent to lower a patient's oestrogen levels for three to five years. My radiation oncologist and I agreed we would delay taking a decision regarding my use of Tamoxifem until my body had recovered from the surgery and the radiation.

It is difficult for me to describe my hassles over the possible use of that drug. One thing soon became absolutely clear, my body, my intuition was insisting I didn't need it. Yet against my body and its intuition was ranged the full weight of current Western medical opinion. Tamoxifem is regarded as a wonder drug: it reduces the size of already existing malignant tumours, minimises the possibility of secondary cancers and has few side effects. What sort of a nut was going to say, "thank you very much, I don't want it?" And, if two years hence I were to develop a secondary cancer, how would I live with myself and the dismay of Ian and my family.

Sleepless night has followed sleepless night. I consulted my trusted group of friends: each illuminated a particular aspect of the problem. "It's a battle between the left and right hemispheres of your brain," said Rob, "a battle between your rational, logical, conscious mind and your bodily intuition." It helped, but did not resolve the impasse, to see it in those terms. "You are being asked to live by your professional beliefs," said Leith, my artist friend. True also.

I do believe that all illness has some basis in the psyche, so that at some level cancer has some emotional roots. Ever since I had the diagnosis I have been working with Jennifer; we are fairly confident I have identified the emotional issues. So that on my terms there ought to be no relapse no secondary cancer for me. But as my dear, logical, rational husband says, "Can you ever be sure you have identified all the emotional issues?" And in terms of absolute certainty, no, of course I can't. So why does that childhood incident in the sleep-out keep popping into my mind? What is it trying to tell me?

Let's go back, a small girl asserts herself against a hitherto trusted authority figure and as a result the relationship ends painfully and abruptly. She tries to tell her mother, another authority figure, and is told she is wrong, leading to these life-long ghostly feelings of uncertainty as to the correctness of her own views, as I have described earlier. This was a nasty place to be and affected our small girl in a number of ways. She couldn't handle anger in personal relationships. She was constantly fearing rejection by those to whom she offered affection. Trust was impossible. She would do almost anything for harmony. She hated fuss, confusion and uncertainty. Having once asserted herself to protect herself with such disastrous consequences, she becomes the epitome of Mummy's good girl.

There are actually two issues here, aren't there? One is simply the need to assert myself to protect myself; the other, the possibility that such an assertion may put me alone and unsupported out in the cold. So, finally, I understood: the Tamoxifem issue was so difficult because it was forcing me to consider standing against authority, refusing the drug therapy, defying mainstream medicine and alienating most of my family and friends. Ian, I knew, would be devastated if the oncologist recommended the drug and I refused.

These two issues of assertion and the risk of the cold are central to my cancer saga as I have experienced it. As I have been writing this letter I have wondered if I am merely restating the feelings I unearthed in the last. On reflection, I think not. In daring me, goading me to act in a way that is contrary to age-old feelings, my intuition is forcing me to go beyond the behaviour of those people who discover their issues and then simply chatter about them.[95] It is coercing me, in fact, to take responsibility for my own life in a possible life and death situation.

Yes, I am intelligent, well educated and articulate; I appear quite capable of a simple act of assertion. Yet I know that if the consequences are to be confusion about right and wrong, a consequent lack of harmony and a feeling of being alone and unsupported, being out in the cold, I find myself all but paralysed. This episode, however, says that irrespective of the consequences, I have to face the challenge of exercising my own power and taking responsibility for my own life.

Once I saw it in those terms, my course of action became clear, even if I still found the action itself extremely difficult. So I made my negotiating plan, marshalled my arguments and went to see the oncologist prepared to do battle. "Well," he said, looking up, "people such as you with a small tumour in the first stage of development have an 80%-90% chance of surviving the next five years." (The life span of any remaining existing cancer cell.) "So with odds that good why run the risk of the side effects of Tamoxifem?" Why indeed! All my hassles, all that angst, all my planning and then I am offered exactly what my body says it needs! No Tamoxifem. I accepted gratefully.

Ian and I went for coffee after my appointment. "Oh," he said quietly, "I am so relieved he didn't recommend Tamoxifem. I knew you

---

95 See *Owning and Honouring*, p. 70

didn't really want to take it and I knew I would be very upset if you didn't." I could only agree.

It wasn't all for nothing, though, Friend, was it? I had to be forced to see where my inability to assert myself was leading. This is an old boot; a repressed feeling which I was able to see reflected in the depths of the mirror once I stayed sufficiently still, once I accepted myself. I can't say I enjoyed this view of myself — my tendency to appease in the interests of harmony.

Yet I know there are advantages in facing the shadow. We repress emotions because they brought us such pain as children. That pain makes us regard those feelings as bad, or unwanted. As adults, however, we may need those feelings. Moreover, used in conjunction with the rational mind and adult balance, they may not be negative at all.

This is clearly the case with assertion. All adults, male and female, young and old need to be able to assert themselves in order to be able to protect themselves. I cannot expect other people to protect me. And, in any event, only I really know myself and my own needs. Assertion doesn't necessarily mean going out in the cold; but, if it does, that is the price to be paid for self-protection. It seems I needed the trauma of breast cancer to goad me into daring to use my own power to protect myself irrespective of the consequences.

Yet, look what I have set up as I have been writing. Much of this cancer saga has been about acceptance, the need to accept the nasties of this life, what the Universe doles out to us, to trust that somehow we will be all right. And now I am writing of an equally powerful feeling, to be able to assert oneself, to protect oneself. How am I to reconcile these two? How can I know when I have to accept and when I have to assert?

I don't know the answer to that fundamental conundrum. I am, though, reminded of a very old prayer about choice and decision-making that was said before every meeting of my school councillors all those years ago. "*God grant me the courage to change those things that must be changed, the serenity to accept those things that cannot be changed and the wisdom to know the difference.*" Courage and serenity, what a lovely pair, how do I choose between them? By listening to the wisdom of my body, the depth and intensity of my own intuition and bringing to it all the reliable factual information my conscious mind is able to collect.

It is nine months now since I had my cancer diagnosis, I feel as if I have lived nine years, ninety years, a lifetime perhaps. Maybe now there can be peace in our time.[96]

---

96 Ultimately despite this medical advice and the heeding of my own intuition, to the considerable surprise of all, I was diagnosed with secondary breast cancer affecting my right hip, my lower spine and the outer surfaces of my lungs in February 2002, some eight and a half years after the primary cancer. See *Death as a Friend*, p. 298

'Consider the Lilies in the Field, How They Grow...'

Acceptance Again

For some months I have been here, very quietly at "Binowee", slowly recovering from breast cancer — the ravages of surgery and radiation therapy.

Physically I have been just exhausted: breakfast in bed, a snooze after lunch, and early nights have been the pattern of the day. My only real activity has been to plan the yurt garden. Otherwise my days have been a lazy drift of floating, dreaming, pottering. Mentally, too, I have been very quiet: no Rosen practice, no book writing, no serious reading, not even many letters written. To my great relief the emotional storms occasioned by the radiation have slowly subsided. Now I am dry-eyed for three to four days in a row, that's progress! So on all three levels — the physical, the mental, the emotional — I have been following the wisdom in the phrase "be still".

Generally, I sit down, pen in hand and the words flow. Not this time, this is my third attempt, and still I am stumbling. Is this a product of being still, I wonder? Let me have one last try.

Usually I start with the physical, the particular. A known and trusted technique. Back to basics, then, what has been happening in my body? During these first months since my cancer treatment, I have had much pain all down my right side — my foot, calf, hip joint, buttock, shoulder and arm. I took it both to a masseur here in Tumut and to my trusty acupuncturist in Canberra. We all agreed that this would be the stress of the last few months. My body, it seemed, was releasing the cancer, surgery and radiation therapy in its own way and at its own speed. My role, it seemed, was that of a spectator — in a word acceptance.

In a recent massage session, talking quietly of my life, the phrase *consider the lilies* popped into my mind[97]. The lilies grow, they don't toil, they don't spin; yet Solomon, the greatest, wisest, most splendid of all kings, was not arrayed like one of them. The phrase stayed for days bringing great peace, a relief from the physical pain. The message was clear. Every lily, every flower, every acorn, is in its appointed place in the Divine Garden. So, too, am I, Judith; if I stay quietly where I have been planted, I will grow. I don't have to toil and spin, fret and push; I just have to stay quietly and allow the movement from within. Thus will I acquire my own quiet beauty, whatever that may be.

What is it that differentiates the lily, a rose and an oak tree from me, Judith? It has to be acceptance, doesn't it? The lily never seeks to be other than a lily, so, too the rose, the oak tree. But Judith, ah, Judith... This brings me to a letter I wrote last month. On my overseas trip to see Mark and his family at the end of last year, I had received warm and generous hospitality from a close friend, one whose own life has been fraught with emotional hassles, anger, and at times, violence. I watched my letter of thanks grow, it seemed to write itself, to be addressed to two people, both my friend the recipient, and myself the author. In so far as I was offering unquestioning acceptance of my friend, irrespective of anger, violence or any other nasty, in so far as I offered trust, abiding affection to another, so

---

97 Bible, King James version, Gospel according to *St. Luke*, chapter 12, verse 27.

also was I offering it to myself. Acceptance…

My letter finished, I found that deep within my own psyche I was still, quiet, peaceful, at rest. Possibly for the very first time in my life I was not pulling at myself. I, Judith, was O.K. just exactly as I was. I didn't have to strive to repress bits of myself I would rather not be, nor seek to be something I was not. I wandered into the garden, down to the river; magic was in the air. Words such as respite, cherishing, being be-loved floated up. I, Judith, could offer Judith, comfort, ease, and respite from the constant, ever-present psychological tug of war. I, Judith, could cherish Judith; Judith be-loved of Judith, just exactly as she was, no movement, nothing. Be still... being still, being a lily in the field.

A word of warning about the word acceptance.[98] Often it seems to me to be used with reference to a knuckling down, a bowing before the inevitable with gritted teeth, clenched fists and burdened shoulders. Beneath this so called, apparent, acceptance lies bitterness, resentment, anger, corrosion of the spirit. One is both superficially "accepting" and denying, fighting against the situation; at the same time.

In true acceptance there is no denial. One accepts the inevitable and moves to build it into one's life. It is this latter, making it a part of one's life that is crucial. So, I have had cancer, various consequences follow, these are now an inescapable part of my future. I can deny the situation, rage at it, or, accepting it, make the most of it and see where it leads me. In the same way with the various facets of one's personality that ideally one would rather not have, one can repress them (the Jungian shadow), rage at them, or have a look at them, accept them, and see what they have to offer.

If, as it appeared, I was being offered acceptance of Judith by Judith, then I had to accept the whole situation: there could be no pulling or fretting anywhere. I would have to live my appointed life quietly, gracefully and, if possible, with a touch of humour. Golly it was hard. After a lovely family Christmas here, at "Binowee", with all the children, all the grandchildren, including the two tiny new grandsons born late in 1993 — my Binowee babies — my life became quiet and secluded. I could see my

[98] See *The Mirror of Life*, p. 153 and *The Angel of Pain*, p. 292 for other aspects of acceptance.

future — a little old lady swapping recipes for jam, living vicariously through the doings of her children and grandchildren. I fretted and pulled against being boring, ordinary, dull. Surely, surely, I cried, there must be more to my life than this.

This was my ego speaking. Not only my ego, but all egos. All egos like to be out in front, attracting notice whether by good behaviour or bad. Notice, attention, is the staff of life to egos, there is nothing egos fear so much as being boring, ordinary. Curious what a pejorative word ordinary has become, it seems now to carry overtones of being inferior/mediocre in some way. And yet surely it means standard, normal, natural, usual. My ego was being asked to accept the natural, normal, unremarkable life of a woman of my age slowly recovering from cancer. My ego was so restive: it was weeks, no months, before it began to subside gracefully, to accept the inevitable. This was how life had to be, was meant to be, at least for the moment.

The word ordinary takes me suddenly to thoughts of a lovely spiritual book Ingrid gave me when I left Sweden — *Reflections of an Elder Brother*[99]. In it Bartholemew, the elder brother of the title, states that absolutely everything is part of the Divine, every ant, grain of sand, elephant, space rocket, anything and everything. Over the years, this has become my position too. Thus to be ordinary, an ordinary ant, a space rocket, Judith, is to take one's allotted place as a part of the Divine. In so far as I don't accept that, strive to be extraordinary, different, to be out in front, noticed, I will be acting from my ego needs and in that mode, it appears, I shut out, leave no room for, the designs of the Divine.

Where does all this bring me? Back to my beautiful Goobragandra Valley and my jewel-like "Binowee". Here I find a woman slowly coming to terms with her cancer. She is ordinary in that she is quietly living the life of a convalescing woman of her age. As she goes about her life she probes deeply into her "ordinariness" and discovers ever more depths of an ever increasing richness. There are jewels in those depths. Acceptance was the one I found this time, and with it the peace that passeth all understanding.

---

[99] Joy Franklin and Mary-Margaret Moore (eds), *Reflections of an Elder Brother*, Bartholomew, High Mesa Press, New Mexico, 1990.

PART VIII

Dancing with Death

Then Almira spoke, saying,
We would ask now of death.
And he said:
...life and death are one,
even as the river and sea are one.

...For what is it to die but to stand naked in the wind
and melt into the sun?

Khalil Gibran
The Prophet

Odd Man Out

Tears have always come easily for me, even more so since I did my Rosen training. In 1996, some years after my breast cancer, suddenly they were frighteningly close. I cried every day, for anything and everything. I went to Canberra, walked and talked with Jennifer. "It feels like grief," I said, " but I can't find what I am grieving for." "If you were one of my clients," she replied, "I would suggest a box of tissues and a very sad video: just sit watching, crying and see what comes up."

I was staying with friends in Canberra, a sad video was not an option, but I bought the tissues, and set out in the car for the Cotter River- a hauntingly beautiful and powerful place for me. Suddenly, while I was still driving, the images erupted; overtaken by deep, racking, tearing sobs, I pulled up on the verge.

I saw myself nearly sixty years ago standing in the long thin passage of the house of my childhood. My mother and father rush up and down, in and out, coming and going. "'Bye Babe," from my mother, "'bye Duck," from my father, "take care of yourself, don't do anything I wouldn't do." Another image: I am in my space, the sleep-out. Mum and Dad are there, through that window just on the other side of that wall; but the window is closed, blind down, curtains drawn. There they are, two together in their big warm bed, I have cuddles there in the mornings; but now it is dark, night, and I am out here alone in the cold with my dolls and dear teddy.

Words flash through my mind: I don't belong, have never belonged, no matter what I do, wherever I go, I am always one of three, always the odd man out: a couple and a child, a pair and a child, my parents and a child. Always one child, always alone, always different, always on the outside looking in, no siblings, no peers, no tribe of my own, nowhere I feel I belong.

The operative word here is feeling: not feeling a part of their life, not feeling I belonged, feeling like the odd man out. There was no cruelty here, no neglect, no abuse. My parents were loving, I knew that, but life was busy, pressured: both my grandmothers were ill; one died of breast cancer, her widowed husband came to live with us; my other grandmother had intermittent strokes, she too came to live with us; my father's youngest sister, only eight years older than I, came to live with us. They came in rotation, ours was only a two bed-roomed half a house; each time I went back to the sleep-out. Each time there was more pressure on the house, more pressure on my parents.

When I watched these images, other feelings surfaced, completely hidden for nearly sixty years: I was too much part of their adult life. There I was at grown-up gatherings, alone and watchful on the grown-up edge of the circle; at Saturday tennis sitting and watching; at golf, either walking around, or sitting in the car reading and waiting — I hated that. I was going out with them, helping with guests at home, always a child alone in an adult world. And so, I grew old beyond my years. "Is Judith going to the picnic?" Libby's mother asked. Libby was my closest school friend. "Good, then you may go too, Judith is so sensible!"

As I write now, it does not seem so very important; so I was an only child, so I had no brothers or sisters, so I spent time alone, playing alone, so I spent more time with adults, so what... I know I was greatly loved, grew up in a warm, loving and harmonious household: there were books, music and people. My father was a warm, outgoing man, he was always asking people to tea, drinks, a meal, and later, when we had a beach house, to stay for the weekend. Never had I dreamt that all these unconscious nasties had lurked underneath this known loving warmth. Never could I have imagined the tearing pain of not belonging, being different from, separate from, alienated from, on the outside looking in.

When I looked back down my life, this feeling of not belonging, being different from, separate from, was with me at every level, every turn. Most diplomats never feel they belong to the countries of their overseas assignments: they may speak the language, know the history, the culture, the institutions, but they do not feel that emotional pull that says "this is home." And that is how it should be. Nor do they feel they completely belong in Australia, they are different because they go abroad so regularly. I remember my sister-in-law saying to me once how lucky I was, that with all the coming and going, I did not have to conform. Yes I was lucky, there is freedom in not having to conform; it is though a lonely place to be, on the outside looking in. In any case this freedom is balanced by having to perform on the public stage.

I saw myself in groups of people, at a cocktail party, a school fete, a reunion; I realised I had never felt easy in groups, had always felt in some indefinable way that I did not belong, that the others did not want me. Now I realised all these years later, that these were my feelings, which might not have had any connection to the feelings of others. I also realised how basic, fundamental these feelings were: core feelings, going to the heart of my psyche.

In the ensuing days, flashback followed flashback: I felt the power in the punishments of exile, banishment, ostracism, solitary confinement. To be denied the right to belong cuts deep — "not to belong" is akin to "not to be", I needed to belong somewhere, to establish an identity, a sense of being. No wonder I had felt this obsessive need to be so very good, not only had the Ant suggested that my mother might not return if I was naughty, but now I found I had to be sensible, responsible, good, to deliver to other people whatever it was they wanted. Only thus could I hope to be accepted into someone else's tribe, only thus could I ever hope to belong, to move inside another's magic circle. Yet, where was Judith in all this, what happened to the adventure-loving imp, who might have enjoyed naughtily exploring at the picnic?

Then in September 1996 disaster struck as I became most unwell with a heavy and deep chesty cough. Repeated trips over two months to the doctor, a relatively inexperienced man standing in for my own GP, brought assertions that the tests showed nothing amiss: I had a virus, he said, and later a post viral syndrome. Struggling as I was with unexpected amounts of administrative work involved in the Rosen intensive program, trying to write my book, feeling generally lousy, I was angry with him, frustratedly feeling both unseen and unheard. As it happened most of my usual support network were deeply involved in their own busy lives. Only Ian was there, steady as a rock; together we struggled with my obvious lack of health.

When my own doctor returned in early November, we patiently unravelled the indications of my very obvious ill health. "You know," he said quietly, "sometimes the symptoms you have are indicative of depression. What is going on in your life at the moment?" As he paused, my fury and frustration at my ill health and more particularly the administrative hassles of the burgeoning Rosen program that were depriving me of so much peace and quiet for my writing erupted. We looked at each other, "I will arrange for you to see a specialist physician in Wagga," he said, "but you need to go home and see how you can reorganise your life."

At this point fate intervened. The breast cancer oncologist, whom I had gone to see for a regular check up, sent me for further tests. "I am always uneasy," he said, "when one of my cancer patients has a long lasting apparently inexplicable illness." How right he was. Those tests, together with a follow up bone marrow biopsy, showed acute myeloid leukaemia. I was in hospital having chemotherapy within thirty-six hours, a large question mark over my long-term future.

Suddenly my normal support network reorganised its priorities and materialised as if from thin air. Too ill for most visitors and phone calls, not allowed flowers for fear of germs, I received cards and letters from close friends all round the world. A beautiful kaleidoscope of colours and shapes grew daily on the board on the hospital wall opposite the foot of my bed. I lay watching it, drifting with the names and messages within. The nurses asked about them, we talked of this one and that. It was as if each and every one of those not-physically-present friends was there in the room, holding me steady, as, of course, were Ian and the children, steadying me, steadying one another.

Floating sleepless one night, I saw what happened. Over the years, I had built my own tribe, a group to which I belonged. As an only child, I knew a big family was important to me. Not only did Ian and I have four children, but despite the separations and upheavals of diplomatic life, we are still a close knit and supportive family unit — my tribe. Then there were close friends scattered world wide: friends from overseas postings, Rosen friends, school friends, university friends; people who had touched me in some way, to whom I had offered a piece of myself in return. They too were my tribe, a group to whom I felt I belonged, whom I would support in time of need, as they in turn were rallying to me in my time of need. It was a lovely feeling to be so supported, held so secure, so loved at such a time. To belong — no longer to be the odd man out.

Land of Confusion

What did Kipling say about confusion? Something about keeping your head when all around you were losing theirs? I can't remember exactly, but I can see one thing clearly this morning, I am confused, a feeling I have always disliked. I suppose people who like to "know", as I do, find confusion unsettling. What is happening that confusion hovers? In a word *death*; a simple enough word in itself, but a minefield of confusion.

I have now come to the point where I have to write of having leukaemia, facing the reality of my death in the short term, with a multitude of associated feelings. It was, as you can imagine, a time of great confusion. When I had breast cancer I was still strong enough to continue my daily journal and my regular letters. Thus when I came to write of it some years later, I had my record. However, with my leukaemia, I was far too ill and weak to write for many months and so there is no contemporaneous record. I have some notes I wrote a few months after my last spell in hospital but, wait for it, I now find them confusing!

The sensible thing to do seems to be to start at the beginning. How did all this start? Looking back, I see first a wonderful completely irresponsible holiday that Ian and I had in Europe and southern

Zimbabwe in April-July of 1996. No one was expecting us to do anything, each night we had only to decide how we wanted to spend the next day — pure magic.

On our return to Australia, Gloria Hessellund came from California to conduct the first Rosen Bodywork intensive. To our great delight there were sixteen participants who all said they would be interested in attending another intensive in November. It appeared our intensive program was under way with the possibility that some of the participants would train as Rosen Method Bodywork practitioners. Additionally, the farm, the Yurt, the garden, all our major projects, seemed to be flowing along sweetly. We appeared, in fact, to be heading for a time of peaceful consolidation after some fairly rough years.

Then in September 1996 came my ill health and finally a visit to a specialist haematologist at the Canberra Hospital[100]. His room in the hospital was white and clinical, but at least the sun streamed in. "You have acute myeloid leukaemia (AML)," he said in his quiet compassionate voice, "this is a serious, aggressive cancer of the bone marrow, cancer of the immune system itself. If you don't have any treatment you will die within the next three months; if you have the treatment we can offer, you may live one, three, five years, we really can't tell." The speaker was a tall slender man with grey curly hair and steady eyes, a man I instinctively trusted. "May I call you Michael?" I asked, it seemed important to establish a close relationship since we were going to have to fight for my life together.

My first thought while still in Michael's room was my book. If time was going to be short then nothing else mattered, everything, everyone else would have to move out of my life. I looked across the room at Ian, "My book", I said, "Yes", he confirmed, "your book, you will have to pull through this to finish it." Other people could continue the Rosen training, other people could build a garden, although it would not be the one I would have created. But I had spent ten years researching the body-mind-spirit connection; I alone could write up that material.

It was, I found both stunning and shocking to be told of my very

---

[100] See *Odd Man Out*, p. 253

possible death in the near future. Although my memory of the rest of that interview is hazy, one thing will be engraved on my heart till the day I die, a simply incredible feeling of being stripped absolutely naked — so raw I felt as if I had been skinned.

We were asked to sit in the waiting room while arrangements were made for my immediate admission to hospital. I knew there was no way I could sit with others, have others look at my nakedness, see me so vulnerable, so powerless, so helpless. "Let's just walk quietly up and down the corridor," I said to Ian. So arm and arm, up and down we went, quietly, slowly, soothed by the rhythm of our footsteps. We had lived nearly all our adult lives together, were in fact to celebrate our fortieth wedding anniversary in ten days time. What on earth did life have in store for us now?

AML, we discovered, is treated by drugs that play havoc with the DNA of leukaemic cells in the bone marrow to such an extent that they die. There is a wonderful irony here. Not only was I very ill, weak and confused, but the treatment for my particular illness was more confusion! Little wonder that during those first weeks of treatment it was all but impossible to see any patterns, to gain any idea what meaning this particular experience might have for me. With hindsight, confusion would have to have been the first leitmotif to emerge and this at every level of our lives.

Ian needed somewhere to live in Canberra (friends helped, bless them), yet he also had to keep an eye on the farm in Tumut. The children all wanted to come, all had lives to lead, priorities to rearrange. Invitations had been sent out for Pip's wedding to be held in Melbourne a few days after Christmas. A dressmaker was at that moment cutting out fabric I had bought at Liberty's in London for my dress for the wedding. Would we carry on with the wedding, would I be able to attend? Michael at least had an answer to that one. There was no way my immune system would be strong enough for me to attend a wedding in a marquee in Melbourne with a hundred germ-laden guests, although a small family ceremony in the garden at Tumut might just be a possibility…he would see.

Behind this lay the ever-present issue of death and dying — my death and my dying. Suddenly, this was no longer an intellectual proposition, something we all know will eventually come into our lives, but right in the room with me every minute of every day. What was it about death, I asked myself? Was I afraid of actually dying, the ultimate fear of the unknown? Was I afraid of the process of dying, many people have to live through pain-filled, protracted deaths with much loss of dignity? Or was something else at the core of the grief that had me crying every day.

I don't think I will know whether or not I am afraid of the actuality of death until that moment comes. However, as I write I see myself standing sobbing at the foot of my hospital bed. One of the nurses is holding me, comforting me, asking me what this is all about? I have always loved life passionately, even when it has dealt me some tough cards, I tell her. The thought of it fills me with a wonderful vibrant feeling; I am excited by it, curious about all aspects of it. I just love it. With her gentle help, I discovered it was the thought that my life might soon be coming to an end that was filling me with such a deep and almost inconsolable sense of grief.

That same night a curious fleeting incident occurred. As I searched for the tight places in my body, trying to relax, I came across a tiny spot right in the depths that I had never found before — a spot so sensitive, so subtle, so intangible and yet at the same time very real. As I touched it with a feather like stroke from my mind, a word floated up, soul, my soul. Simultaneously I saw an image of the graph of an innings in a one-day cricket match: a continuous white line representing the innings, black dots at intervals representing the fall of wickets. It sounds way out even for me, but that imagery brought such respite, such comfort. For as I understood it symbolically, that white line was the passage of my soul through eternity, those black dots each life as it was lived. It seemed I need not fear or grieve for the loss of my life. My soul would travel quietly on through eternity; only this physical body would die, once its innings came to an end.

I also found it comforting that life continued despite my illness. Michael agreed we could celebrate our fortieth wedding anniversary picnicking with Pip and two very close friends in the courtyard adjacent to my ward. True I had to wear a hat and mask looking, as Pip remarked, just like a cowboy from a Western. But it was fantastic to be outside and our friends produced a delicious lunch within the limits of my restrictive diet. Later in the afternoon came a surprise visit from the nursing staff, singing happy wedding anniversary to the tune of happy birthday, and bearing a delicious strawberry cream sponge courtesy of the hospital kitchen. We have celebrated our wedding anniversaries all over the world in many different ways. This was one of the most touching and most memorable.

Plans for Pip's wedding progressed also. It was my idea, in the dead of a sleepless night, that we have a very small informal family wedding ceremony on Boxing Day in our garden at Tumut, followed by the already planned "wedding" in Melbourne on the twenty-eighth of December. Since by this time Pip and Stephen would have been legally married all of forty-eight hours, they would reaffirm their vows! Stephen's family generously agreed to the travelling involved and a group of loving friends made the Tumut arrangements. The dress maker contributed, coming to the hospital for fittings and even making me a cloche hat from remaining scraps of silk to soften the appearance of my hair loss. Jill perceptively remarked that the wedding seemed important in showing us that life was going on irrespective of my leukaemia.

Why am I writing of what appear to be the trivialities of my hospital experience? The word that comes to mind immediately is *love*. Never have I felt so loved as I did those first few weeks in hospital. There I was in the High Dependency Unit, ill, weak and frail, minus my hair, of no apparent use to anyone, needing oxygen, blood transfusions, platelet transfusions and a very high degree of skilled nursing care that was given unstintingly and compassionately.

My family and friends also gave of themselves in countless ways. Ian, in particular, apart from brief visits to Tumut to check on the farm, sat strong and comforting in my room for days on end, and even one night when I called for him because I thought I might not be alive in the morning. All the children came regularly to support me, Ian and one another. Somewhere in Sydney lives that generous blood donor who provided additional blood for my rare blood group once my requirements had exhausted the supply in the Canberra Blood Bank. It was the unconditional nature of that love that filled me with such joy. As I lay fighting for my life, love, help and support poured in. When I later remarked to Jennifer that I had been lucky not to have contracted any of the infections that are such a hazard in the treatment of AML, she was most robust in her reply. "Lucky," she said, "no germ had a chance against any one as cocooned in love as you were."

After four weeks in hospital I went home for ten days before returning to hospital to repeat the process.[101] I went home with mixed feelings. It was wonderful to be away from the hospital, and most especially its food.[102] Marvellous to be able to walk freely outside in the garden without the restriction of a mask. Yet the results of a second bone marrow biopsy had shown that five percent of the bone marrow cells were still cancerous. I was often sleepless with a constant image of something black and all-powerful spreading its claws or tentacles through my body, tearing at me, strangling me. I recognised this imagery from my breast cancer — my fear of those remaining cancer cells. It was not nice.[103]

One bad night I took a pull on myself. Surely, I said, after all these years of bodywork, my reading and my own experiences, I must know that my unconscious, through my body, is always trying to help me, trying to show me things about my life I would not otherwise have understood. If this is so, then I have to stop pulling against these remaining cancer cells, listen to my body and try to understand its message. Somehow I have to see

---

101 In 1996 the treatment Michael recommended for my acute myeloid leukaemia comprised three month-long spells in hospital (an induction and two consolidations) in each of which I had a period of intense chemotherapy twenty-four hours a day. The drugs attacked the cancerous cells in my immune system but also the healthy cells. After about two weeks I became what is called neutropenic, someone whose neutrophil count is less than 0.5. Since neutrophils (one of the white blood cells) are the body's first line of defence against infection, my immune system was incapable of protecting me. Regular transfusions of haemoglobin and platelets kept my bone marrow ticking over and regular intravenous doses of antibiotics gave me some protection.

Finally the healthy cells from my immune system started to function again and strengthen to the point where it was safe for me to leave the hospital and go home for a short rest before returning to repeat the process. It was a gruelling process both physically and emotionally.

102 I lived in a single room, on a diet which prohibited uncooked fruit or vegetables and any food containing a living culture. I was now only strong enough to see the immediate family and a few close friends in good health. No flowers were permitted (possible germs in the water), and, if I left my room I had to wear a mask. Pneumonia was the dread. If I should be so unlucky as to contract it I would probably die.

103 See *On Being Squeezed*, p. 230 My unconscious chose the same imagery in both cancers.

leukaemia as positive — life giving — rather than negative physical life destroying — otherwise I am virtually asking it to bring my life to a close.

Since leukaemia is a disease of the bone marrow, deep in the core of the body, in terms of the body-mind continuum it must be pointing to a lack of ease, an imbalance deep in the core of the psyche.[104] Some quiet reflection showed me that in being so "good"[105] and meeting the expectations and values of others, in order to belong to a tribe,[106] I was not necessarily living my own life. In the simplest terms this was a terminal illness for my psyche. My soul had come into being in order to live its own unique life, fulfil its own particular potential, anything else was a living death.

Thus my insight that night was that this cancer had come to offer me the freedom to live my own life and to do some of the things that were important to me. I had to face it; I was not subject to a demanding and tyrannical family, nor abusive friends and work colleagues. Ian, in particular, had always been openly and deeply supportive of my attempts to develop my own interests.This need to meet the expectations of others was mine, fuelled by experiences in my own unconscious. I needed to deal with it or I would surely die of leukaemia.

Gae is a lovely woman who lives further up our valley. She was here the morning after this insight helping to prepare the house for the influx of visitors at Christmas and for Pip's wedding."How are you feeling?" she asked. I told her of my insight the previous night. "Yes," she said, "I thought something must have happened, you look so much better this morning."

The Universe was kind, the twilight for Pip and Stephen's wedding was clear crisp, not too hot.The garden looked lovely, as did we all. It was such a happy, loving, family occasion, dear God, let's hope it was a good omen for many more to come.

[104] See *A Broader Canvas*, p. 159

[105] See *Bendigo*, p. 101

[106] See *Odd Man Out*, p. 253

The Mystery of Life

Dear Friend,

If the leitmotif of my first spell in hospital was confusion, that of my second would have to be trust, trust at every level. A few days before returning to hospital for my second spell, I had a bizarre experience. Lying quietly in bed one night, I suddenly saw chemotherapy as a metaphor for sexual union. The "induction" (that first dose of drugs) as the union between a male lover and his young virgin female partner. Although that young virgin was apparently open and trusting, she later realized the extent to which she had been unconsciously holding back, protecting herself.[107]

Do you remember how terrified I was of the possibility of chemotherapy during my breast cancer? With the leukemia diagnosis, I had shocked both Ian and myself by saying that I felt so dreadful I simply wanted to fall into a hospital bed and have "chemo". Initially, I was frightened; however, once the nurses assured me the drugs were safe in my blood stream, I tried to see the whole process positively and open myself both physically and psychologically to the healing being offered. Yet, as I watched that imagery that night at home, I realised the extent to which I had held back during that first spell of chemotherapy.

Now, my intuition was saying, during this second spell, if the drugs are to have a chance to purify my body totally, my whole being must be absolutely still, quite flat as it were, in order to allow them to penetrate every tiny fibre of my being. There must be complete trust, absolute openness, no holding back.

It was such a relief to talk regularly with Jennifer about my feelings, my dreams, and the imagery floating up from my unconscious. When next we spoke she took me deeper into my unconscious. "Don't forget," she said, "that sexual union between two people deeply in love and wholly committed to one another, releases transforming energies deep

---

[107] See *On Being Squeezed*, p. 230 for a similar experience during my radiation therapy for breast cancer.

within the psyche." She paused for a minute, "And if we continue that metaphor," I replied, "the chemotherapy drugs will also be deeply transforming, so long as I am able to be absolutely open to them."

The nurses and doctors had all suggested that my second spell in hospital would be less stressful than the first. This was quite correct. I knew the procedures this time; I also knew the hospital routine and the nursing staff. There was less fear of the unknown, less panic as to what might happen to me; fewer feelings of powerlessness or helplessness. In short there was at least a modicum of trust. In metaphoric terms the virgin had survived her wedding night. Trust seemed to be the issue.

It surfaced initially around the writing of this book. During my Rosen training I began my letters to you, my collection of unposted letters to a friend.[108] Slowly it became apparent I had the makings of a book. Once I returned to Australia, in late 1991, I saw myself more clearly as researching in my own body and my own unconscious the connection between the body, the mind and the spirit. A connection I could also see as I worked with my clients and participants in Rosen intensives.

However, fate seemed to intervene every time I started to write my book. Ian had a mystery virus (possibly from time in Papua New Guinea) and was in hospital for some weeks; he then came off his horse and broke five ribs; I had breast cancer and was unable to write for fifteen months; finally I had been swept up in the detailed administration of the recently commenced Australian Rosen intensive program. To my immense frustration the book always seemed to be on the back burner, just out of reach.

During my second spell in hospital a niggle about my book surfaced. Maybe, I thought to myself, I unconsciously permit other things to interrupt the writing because I am frightened that the project is not worthwhile, or, more likely, that I won't be able to manage it. Heigh ho, this was the old childhood pattern of inadequacy surfacing again. No doubt some deeply engrained patterns die a very slow death. It was also, as I quickly saw, a lack of trust in myself, both in my ideas, and in my ability to put them across.

[108] See *Walking in the Woods*, p. 63

Seeking clarity, I asked a close author friend the personal characteristics required for writing a book; endurance and the ability to withstand solitude, was his reply. Suddenly I saw myself with new eyes. Yes I had endurance, I had had treatment for both breast cancer and leukaemia; and yes I could endure solitude. Had I not lived these last ten years without communicating many of my partially formed ideas on the interdependence of the body-mind-spirit. Perhaps I was better equipped to write a book than I had hitherto thought.

"How will you feel if you don't write your book?" asked one of the nurses. To my own surprise I heard myself say, "Oh, I will be saddened, for I will know that I have let myself down." So if I don't trust myself to carry out my own ideas, I let myself down. Of course, it's quite simple if you put it like that. And, put another way, I don't fulfil my potential, and I don't live out my destiny.

A vivid life-like dream brought another aspect of trusting. I saw a woman with a third eye in the middle of her forehead — a well-known symbol of intuition, enlightenment and age-old wisdom. It appeared I knew this woman, recognised her from way back; yet I did not recall that we had ever previously met. Moreover, when she greeted me and said she was a long-time friend, I rejected her saying I did not know her and that she should leave. She was insistent, but I was also. Finally as she left she said she would return. In psychological terms the woman in my dream would be part of myself. With her third eye, she would seem to be a wise woman, my wise old woman. But, I had sent her away. It appeared I could not, or would not, integrate her into my psyche at the moment. So, I would not, or could not, trust myself.

And so day succeeded day, my blood counts dropped, "bottomed out" as the phrase went, and then gradually recovered. Most of this spell in hospital I had the strong intuition that in some way I was going to be all right, whatever that phrase might mean. I think at the time I took it to mean that I would not die in the short term.

Then, as I left the hospital for another break, I had a disturbing conversation with Michael. I thought I had asked him a question about the further treatment required; I think he thought I had asked him about my future. I cannot now remember the exact words he used, but however he phrased them, I took them to mean that my treatments were merely buying me time, that a recurrence was inevitable and that a leukaemia-free future was unlikely. I was deeply disturbed.

My intuition, for which read my wise old woman, is saying that I am going to be all right. On the other hand when my doctor, a male authority figure, gives the classic Western medical response to a leukaemia diagnosis, what do I do? Do I listen to my own body, trust my own intuition, pay attention to my own wise old woman? No, I allow myself to become deeply confused and unhappy; almost as if I lie down and prepare to die. One thing is very clear; at that time trust in myself and my wise old woman were as far away as ever.

The next ten-day spell at home was not a happy time. It was late January, hot, very hot, with temperatures in the mid to high thirties centigrade. Since Ian was only home for about thirty-six hours each week whenever I was in hospital, the house and garden were inevitably beginning to show signs of our long absence. I felt so weak, so very helpless and frustrated. Our lovely garden was overgrown with weeds and in need of constant water. Ian didn't have the time nor I the strength to do much about it. We felt trapped, trapped by my leukaemia and its treatment, trapped by life itself and what it was handing us.

Trapped would have to describe how I felt psychologically. Intellectually I knew I had to come to terms with uncertainty, had to learn to live only in the present moment of each day, simply had to learn to trust. Saying that is one thing, feeling it, living it, is a different matter. I went round and round in circles. During that spell at home I was moody and even closer to tears than usual. I must have been difficult to live with.

Finally during my third spell in hospital relief arrived. I awoke to some of the nastiest pain I ever remember, over my right eye, up through my skull, down behind my right ear and then into my right shoulder — basically the path of the gall bladder meridian in Chinese medicine. My naturopath friends and I suspected this was my liver-gall bladder complaining of the toxins in the "chemo" drugs. In despair I tried to write my journal hoping to steady myself and possibly gain some insights. As I wrote I finally saw that, rather than accepting this pain, looking to see what my body might be trying to tell me, I was fighting, thrashing futilely like a hooked fish. And so I asked myself a classic bodyworker's question, what is this pain about? The answer 'Leukaemia': I was not accepting the pain of having leukaemia, not at all levels.

If I continued, and asked myself what was the pain of leukaemia, for the disease itself is not physically painful, then what would I reply? The answer I gave was the doubt and confusion over my future. I didn't know whether I was going to live one year, three, or five, die of leukaemia or die of other natural causes. I didn't know, can't know and it drives me nearly mad. Logically, practically, intellectually, none of us knows — I understand that. However, I am actually living, feeling every minute of that unknowing; it is that which is pounding in my head, and it is the hardest and most painful thing I have experienced.

This is the ever-curious woman, the scholar, with her burning almost obsessive need to know. This time there can be no knowing; it is an impossibility. Somehow she is going to have to accept that she cannot know and learn to trust, or she will make herself ill. For this particular personality, this is a core issue, isn't it? The need to know, hard up against the impossibility of knowing, bringing into play the necessity of trust.

Over the years, when I am in tough places I ask for Grace. When I do this I simply say quietly to myself, "I am absolutely stuck, I don't know what to do, I can't stand it any longer, please help." I never ask for a particular outcome, for then the ego is involved for its own ego ends. I can't tell you if I ask for help from within, or without. All I know is that if I ask in this way from the depths of my being, I am never refused. So on one very bad night I quietly asked for Grace.

Sure enough some time later an insight floated up. Leukaemia is a disease at the core of the body and affects the immune system, the core of life. Right up against that core of my life I found uncertainty. By a strange coincidence at that same time, some one to whom I was close was battling the uncertainties of becoming pregnant. There was no physical impediment, fertility drugs had been taken; but conception had not occurred. Again uncertainty. Just as the ending of a life is uncertain, so too there is never certainty as to the coming into being of new life.

I have used the words certainty and uncertainty which describe very mundane processes. What I saw that night was that the core of life was a mystery, and this was where I was, hard up against the mystery of life. The Mystery of Life — for that is what it is. Our coming into being, our continued existence, the extinguishing of life, all happen beyond our control. Michael could be correct, I could have recurring bouts of leukaemia, or I could not. In the event I could still die tomorrow as a result of falling under a bus. I don't know, more importantly, I can't know.

It was the phrase Mystery of Life that finally brought relief. I stopped thrashing on my line, stopped seeking the unseekable, and set about the task of adapting to this new way of life. All my life I have been very curious. I don't think I seek knowledge for power, or money or status, I just like to know, have in fact an almost obsessive need to know. So to accept that I have come to the place where no further knowledge is possible is a big step, a very big step indeed.

Later I was to read Matthew Fox's view that with the scientific discoveries of the eighteenth and nineteenth centuries and the great strides in twentieth century research, the concept of mystery has largely disappeared — all mysteries now being regarded simply as unsolved problems.[109] Look at the society in which we live with it's recurring themes of royal commissions, inquiries, reports, research, investigative journalism — all presupposing that we can know, if only we put the correct procedures in place. Where in all of this is the time and the place for awe at the complexity, the wonder of life itself, the magic of life, the Mystery of Life?

---

109 Mathew Fox, *The Coming of the Cosmic Christ*, Harper &Row, San Francisco, 1988

It seems odd, Friend, that confusion with its lack of clarity and order, has always bothered me, made me anxious and even angry; and yet, I have always loved mysteries, secrets and surprises. Maybe it is that these latter intrigue me, spike my curiosity in some way. I am not sure. If I pause, it is also odd that having written so much of my fear of the unknown I should now find respite from the uncertainties surrounding my death by calling them the Mystery of Life. Odd or not, it seems I have to accept it, for that it appears, is how I am.[110]

Finally, during that spell in hospital, I realised I was being asked trustingly to "live" that most fundamental question of all. Put another way, I understood that if only I could stop being so obsessed with needing to know and start to trust both the Universe and myself, I was being offered a chance to live experiencing the wonder, the awe and the magic of my life.

No doubt about it, leukaemia raises many tough questions.

110 See *Kath Wyatt's Daughter*, p. 277

Riding the Tiger

Accepting the Challenges of Life

Dear Friend,

After my first spell in hospital I wrote of confusion, and after the second of trust. This time I find I am a prey to my ambivalence around the effort required to regain my health. Can I find the strength to recover my strength, as it were?

I saw this first in the break between my second and third spells in hospital. Having supper in a restaurant with Ian and watching the diners around me enjoying a lovely summer's evening, I was brought close to tears by feelings of isolation. These people were presumably chatting of their everyday lives: the weather, the food, work, kids, a parking fine. In contrast, my everyday life was about survival: together with everybody else in the oncology ward, I was fighting for my life. I felt as if I had just come back from the trenches, or the mined paddy fields of Vietnam. Would I ever be able to relate to people on an ordinary level again, live a normal life again, I wondered? And just as importantly, where would I find the strength to make the effort?

I was warned that my blood counts would recover more slowly after the third spell of chemotherapy. And so it was. They would rise one day, only to drop the next: one step forward, one step back. It was as if my immune system was saying, "If you are going to continue to treat me with all these toxic drugs, I am not sure it is worthwhile making the effort to recover, I think I might just give up." As the blood counts fluctuated and the days passed, I began to feel as if I would never be able to return home.

When I asked my unconscious what this fluctuation might be reflecting — ambivalence, hesitation — were the words that floated up. I was, my insight suggested, deeply ambivalent about my future. Did I have the courage to leave the care and support of the hospital, signal to my family and friends that I no longer needed such a high level of support and make the tremendous effort required in order to pick up the threads of my life again? And, more fundamentally, did I want to make that effort, if only to find myself a few years down the track with recurring leukaemia? Of one thing I was absolutely certain: I felt utterly incapable of making any effort in any situation.

A would-be helpful visiting friend remarked that a friend of hers had had similar leukaemia to mine and was doing so well — she had suffered only one relapse in three years! I listened aghast. Did she have any idea what she was saying? Only one relapse in three years. So in the space of that three years she would have had six bouts of chemotherapy with all its associated upheavals. What about the quality of her life, was no one considering that?

Although I found that conversation upsetting, it had the unexpected affect of lessening my ambivalence and provoking me into making choices about my future. I had no conceivable interest, I realised, in living my life as a prisoner of leukaemia and its treatments: in and out of hospital, fearing a relapse, having chemotherapy and recovering from the rigours of the cure. I wanted a full vital vibrant leukaemia-free life for however long or short a period. I was not interested in the quantity of my life, only the quality. Without that quality, I did not want to live at all.

Writing to you of the Mystery of Life, I saw it present at the beginning and end of a life. I saw I had to accept that I could have no power at those times and would have to learn to trust.[111] That leaves open the question of my power over my continuing life between those two points, doesn't it? During my third spell in hospital I lay floating with this question. How much power or control over my life do I really have?

Slowly two things became apparent. Jennifer and I had agreed that leukaemia was about transformation, providing me with opportunities to progress beyond recognised former painful childhood patterns, if only I had the courage to grasp them. It was clearly within my power to be

[111] See *The Mystery of Life*, p. 265

"good" on fewer occasions, to meet the expectations of others less, to consider my own values as well as those of the people to whose tribe I wished to belong and to attempt to feel judged or rejected less often. Not only did I have that power; I was, in fact, the only person who did. All I needed was the courage to accept my power and to be responsible for my own life. There could be no feelings of powerlessness or helplessness and no sense of victimisation. Since acting this way would bring feelings of strength, I would not be conscious of effort. Totally exhausted as I was, the possibility of life without effort seemed almost too good to be true.

No matter how strong I become psychologically, I still have no control over the eruption of any "nasties" into my life — cancer, multiple sclerosis or a crippling car accident for instance. I know, from hearing the leukaemia diagnosis, how easily such events bring feelings of powerlessness. Yet, looking back at the months of my treatment, I now see that I chose to use the incredible level of support offered to me, and my own interest in the power of the unconscious, to try to turn my situation around. At the very least, it seems, it is within my power to choose my reaction. And again, this power is uniquely mine. These are the same thoughts I had on first moving to Tumut. Leukaemia, in the same way as the move to Tumut, is capable of giving me more freedom in my life, but with that freedom comes the necessity to make choices for which I will be responsible.[112]

Some weeks after I left hospital for the last time, I went to Canberra to participate in the sharing at a Rosen intensive. It seemed important to talk of how I saw my future, since leukaemia had made my participation in the on-going Rosen program uncertain. Quietly and firmly I shared my desire for a full and vital life irrespective of its length. As I spoke, I could feel the power in what I was saying, feel a shift as my fears of recurrent bouts of leukaemia eased and feel the strength to handle my post-leukaemia life flowing in. It was as if I was making an affirmation to the Universe — "This is how it will be." It was a beautiful few minutes.

---

112 See *The Faces of Freedom*, p. 171

It's easy, though, isn't it, to make an affirmation of how I want things to be? Somehow I still have to learn to apply that thought to the living of my everyday life. While I was still grappling with this issue, the refrigerator in the Yurt broke down a few hours before a party of six were expected to arrive to stay for a week. I was almost overwhelmed — was there never to be an end to the dramas in our life. A stream of thoughts ran through my mind: I just don't want to know about this — flight; followed by who should I ring, what was I going to do, what is going on that everything keeps going wrong — fight? Flight or fight, two usual reactions to any crisis, large or small, both life-saving in the short term, but not supplying long term answers. I can't be continually fighting or fleeing. I had to move from the familiar reaction to the response I should make, which was mine to choose.

The refrigerator was under guarantee. I pulled myself together and rang the supplier. "Michael," I said, "we have a problem" and explained the situation. Without a moment's pause, he replied, "Not a problem, Judith, just a challenge, leave it with me, let me see what I can do." Look at the power of the word: I say *problem*, he says *challenge* and as I listen I sense my feelings change. If it was a problem, given my life at the moment, it was all just too much; but if it was a challenge well, I could probably handle it. In fact as we were speaking, I realised I actually enjoy a challenge. And much more importantly, Friend, look what happens: suddenly, one of my most deeply held negative and limiting feelings — the I can't-cope-syndrome — shifts.[113] I am no longer bedevilled by those limiting, incapacitating feelings.

This is taking me back to the Yogis. It is another application of their view that pain is in the mind.[114] If I can manage to change my thoughts about any situation, then I have in fact the power to change that situation. Well that's a challenge in itself.

The word challenge brings to mind the imagery in Robert Dessaix' beautiful book, *Night Letters*. His hero, making the shocking discovery that he is HIV positive, initially sees the choices for his future life as fight or flight. He could fight the diagnosis and the disease, or he could

[113] See *The Stigmata*, p. 97

[114] See *The Angel of Pain*, p. 292

pretend none of it was happening. After some months of reflective wandering, he says: "I neither faced the lion nor kept on running — I leapt onto its back, stuck a hat on my head and rode off on it. I rode it. Yes, it's true, with my heart in my mouth, but also with true exultation."[115]

After I read this book, the phrase "riding the tiger" surfaced in my mind, grabbing me with such gripping intensity it clearly had a place in my life. It's another aspect of acceptance. You know when I first started my journey, I saw myself seeking freedom. Yet gradually over the years, it has become clear that, paradoxically, acceptance is an integral part of being free — the quiet courage, the serenity, to accept those things I cannot change, be it myself or the challenge of an immutably difficult situation.[116]

Moreover, as I now understand, my acceptance needs two modes. In one, I am still, trying not to exacerbate an already difficult situation by pulling away, twisting from it — Ingrid's *forsoning*.[117] The other contains more movement as I pick up the challenge of a difficult situation and run with it.[118] Ride off into the unknown on my unruly tiger as it were. Well, that's where I am going now — off into the unknown of life after leukaemia with all its hazards, all its challenges.

Thank you my Friend for your support.

---

115 Robert Dessaix, *Night Letters*, Macmillan, Sydney, 1996, p. 272

116 See *Tamoxifem*, p. 241

117 See *Angel of Pain*, p. 292

118 See *Tamoxifem*, p. 241

Kath Wyatt's Daughter

Why, why do I have to keep moving all the time? What have I done to deserve this? And, the last and most bitter question of all, why when after so many moves, so much re-establishing myself in places not of my choosing, did the circumstances of my life manoeuvre me into having to *choose* to leave my beloved "Binowee" in Tumut, one of only two places on this earth where I have felt I really belong. These last few months have been tough.

We were on holiday in Queensland in mid 1999, when Ian remarked quietly one night that he was not sure how much longer he could continue to live in Tumut. Owning a farm, he said, had been one of the things he had always wanted to do. It had initially been a challenging adventure and great fun, but lately it had become a heavy burden that he was not sure he could continue to carry. His bout of cancer and his operation the previous year had been very debilitating.

My heart sank, these were fateful words, although not altogether unexpected. I knew we were no longer the same people as those who had arrived up the Goobra in December 1991. Then we were young, at least in spirit, with all the confidence and enthusiasm of youth for our new life, free for the first time from the constraints of the Department of Foreign

Affairs and Trade. Now, not only were we eight years older, but very much sadder and wiser, with much of our confidence in life and our physical fitness depleted by the rigours of cancer, its treatments and consequent psychological upheavals.

So I knew I had to listen to Ian; he is the loving and much loved partner of my life. If he said he could no longer manage the farm then we would have to move again. Yet it hurts so much — never did I imagine that a piece of land, my "Binowee", could have such power. I am, I discover, as attached to it as to a deeply loved and treasured friend, and my heart is aching as at the death of such a friend, and I actually had to choose to bring this grief on myself…

Let's pause here. What is fuelling this grief? What was so very special about "Binowee" on the banks of the Goobra that brings tears to my eyes as I write, even now some fifteen months later? It seems to be beyond words, and yet we both know I find it difficult to move forward unless I have some glimmer of an understanding of what is holding me back. The unexpected word that floats up as I write is *miracle* — finding and creating the beauty that became "Binowee" was our own small miracle.

The words "Tumut" and "retreat cottage" had first surfaced in my meditation in the 1980s. At that time we knew little of rural living, farming, building and organising a guest cottage, designing and constructing a garden on such a scale. Yet, after Ian retired in 1991, we had followed my meditation and bit by bit everything fell into place. Eight years later, we had an enclave of such beauty that all who came were touched by it in some way. It is curious, you know I never actually felt as if "I" had done it. In fact after the first year or so I did little of the physical labour. My contribution had been the ideas and, yes, if I pause for thought and give credit where it is due, the driving force, the passion behind the project was mine. "Binowee", our small miracle…

So nearly twelve months later we sold that very special property and in mid-2000, moved to the Mornington Peninsula, fifty kilometres south east of Melbourne, in an area also suggested by my meditation. We lived first in Mark and Alice's house, spending three months house hunting before we finally bought and moved into our own home in Mornington itself. It is true we found a lovely, spacious, light, warm house with a most beautiful view over Port Phillip Bay. And yet, and yet, it is unfair, but I do not feel for it as I felt for my Tumut "Binowee". As I write I glimpse a sliver of understanding: am I perhaps grieving for the loss of my involvement in the building of that small miracle? Is that what this is about, I wonder?

We lunched one day with my oldest school friend who had spent many happy school holidays with our family. "Let's go to Flinders," she said, "back to our old haunts". We had heard my parents' house at Flinders was awaiting demolition and so we found it. That was not the best afternoon of my life either. There was the original "Binowee", uninhabited, an empty dilapidated shell, peeling paint, unhinged shutters, drooping gutters and an overgrown, neglected garden; and it had been such a warm, happy, vibrant house in its day. I spoke to one of the neighbours who had been watching us from her garden. I was not a vandal, I said, just Kath Wyatt's daughter come to have one last look at her house.

The following day Ian and I went to meet the eighty-year-old vendor of the house we had agreed to buy. As we were introduced, he greeted me warmly, kissing me on the cheek. "I am told you are Kath Wyatt's daughter," he said, "I used to play golf with your mother. I am so happy to be selling you my beautiful house for I am sure you will look after it for me." Sadly and anxiously he was moving into a retirement village, most uncertainly I was moving after forty odd years back to the outskirts of Melbourne. It was a lovely meeting for both of us convincing me, if nothing else, that this was the house into which we were supposed to be moving.

As we established ourselves in Mornington, I was weepy and borne down by the muddle and confusion of these latest two moves, saying to Ian, that they were just two moves too many, making a total of twenty-two in our forty-four years of married life. So what happened to the woman who wrote to her friend of riding the tiger when she was recovering from leukaemia, who discovered she enjoyed picking up the challenge of difficult situations and building them into her life?[119] Gone into hiding apparently; she was certainly not available to help me cope with those moves.

Yet acceptance still has to have a place. Somehow I have to come to terms with the move from Tumut and the many changes it has brought. How do I move forward, if not by accepting the challenge implicit in difficult situations? Struggling with almost chronic bladder infections not long after my arrival, I talked to an acupuncturist friend. It seemed, I said, as if for some reason the waters of my life were stagnant and therefore germ-laden. This was fanciful and yet helpful. For as we talked of stagnant and associated words such as still and motionless, we made a connection with acceptance. "In accepting", he said, "you seem to see yourself as either motionless or riding your tiger overcoming adversity." That gave pause for thought. "Yes," I said slowly, "although that is an oversimplification of my position, there is something in what you say."

Later that night the word *harmony* floated into my mind with that gripping intensity I have come to associate with my unconscious. Harmony, what did I mean by harmony, and what part could it play in helping me to adapt to my current life? I saw it first in its most obvious, musical context: my mother at the piano, my own piano playing, my love of Bach, Mozart and Beethoven with their clear ordered melodies.

What else did I know of harmony? My dictionaries both stressed that a congruent orderly whole with an absence of friction was the essence of harmony. I found this a colourless mundane description for a word that was beginning to fill me with wonder. As the days passed I had only to think of the word harmony to have my body sing in some way. Clearly there were unconscious, possibly mystical associations here of which I was not yet aware.

In *Riding the Tiger*, I distinguished between being still and riding off on a challenge.[120] Now I began to wonder did Ingrid and I mean still in the sense of stagnant, when we spoke of being "at–one"? Surely not.[121] We had agreed there was to be no movement "away from", not that there was

119 See *Riding the Tiger*, p. 272

120 See *Riding the Tiger*, p. 272

121 See *Angel of Pain*, p. 292

to be no movement at all. Similarly when I ride my tiger I am moving, but again not "away from", for if I pull (move away from the tiger) I fall off. So the issue then, is not movement of itself, but a movement away from.

What happens if I introduce the idea of harmony — bringing with it connotations of the orderly whole — into these ideas of acceptance? So I move, but as a part of a whole in an orderly easy manner. I have just realised where this might be taking me. As I write I see this image of myself, there I am woven into my place in the tapestry that is my life. As that tapestry moves, I move with it. I move in accordance with the Divine plan for the whole, not according to my own ego ends. The problem with the notion of riding a tiger is that it is too simple. It allows space for the ego to say, "look at me, look at what I am doing with this difficulty in my life." In true acceptance of the difficulties in life, the ego needs to bow to the demands of the Divine Unknown at the core of all our lives. So harmony seems to bring with it ideas of moving slowly, easily, patiently and trustingly. Patience and trust would seem to be crucial. Once more we seem to have arrived at living the question.[122]

As the days passed the word harmony began to move into other areas of my life. Thinking of my mother at the piano took me back to other memories of my childhood. Yes, there had been anger at times, and all the stresses of World War II, but in essence ours was a happy, ordered, loving family — harmonious in a word. Suddenly it was as if that one word harmony described my search these last thirteen years. It began to appear that in all my unconscious travels, all my exploration, unknowingly I had been seeking harmony; harmony within myself, harmony in all my dealings with my outer world and harmony in dealing with the crises of my life. And the roots of this search were my overall unconscious memories of such a happy harmonious family childhood.

To see my journey afresh in terms of a search for harmony is not to deny the insights of the last thirteen years. Each of those continues to have its own place in this story. Finding harmony is simply an example of the spiral nature of unconscious travel.[123] My unconscious has moved me

---

[122] See *The Mystery of Life*, p. 265

down another level to another more pervasive feeling that I experience lying beneath my sensitivity, my need to be good, to fulfil the expectations of others, to belong and even possibly to feel that I am wrong. Each of those feelings helps me create a harmonious atmosphere and that it appears is how I most want to live.

When I set out on my travels I wrote, naively as I now see, that I was seeking freedom.[124] Writing of my Rosen training and experiences in Sweden, I realised that to understand how I had experienced my childhood, allowed self-knowledge. This in turn lead to compassion for myself and gradually to freedom from being hassled by my unconscious self and ultimately to self-acceptance. Simultaneously, of course, it was also very gradually permitting me to live in harmony with myself, to live in an ordered, trusting friction-free relationship with myself.

Then, when we went to Tumut, as we developed both the property and the Australian Rosen program, I came to understand that freedom involves the challenges of choice and responsibility. Looking back, harmony seems to play two roles here. First, when I struggled to find a balance between the demands of my would-be clients, the Rosen intensive program and my writing. Secondly, and equally as important, when it says to me that my choices must be exercised responsibly having in mind both my own needs and those of my family and the community in which I live.[125]

Next came the cancer sagas with their grim lessons that the unpredictable disasters of this world erupt into anyone's life and have to be dealt with. At this point I am manoeuvred into accepting the immutable is an integral part of freedom — that paradoxically without acceptance there can be no freedom. If I can accept and then move forward, quietly, patiently and trustingly, then I can live harmoniously in my world and that is what I most want. Finally now all these years later, I am brought to understand that my desire to live a life of harmony is a jewel that lies buried deep in the depths of my unconscious.

More recently I have discovered that some of my feelings are logically inconsistent. I am afraid of the unknown, yet I love mysteries and the

[123] See *The Witchdoctor*, p. 22

[124] See *I Chose Freedom*, p. 39

[125] See *Owning and Honouring*, P. 70

chance to explore. There is my old cannot cope syndrome, and yet we now know I am excited by challenges. It is now beginning to appear that there are mysterious depths in my unconscious, depths where I will not travel. Here lies the Mystery of Life, and that place where all of these apparently inconsistent feelings can be accommodated harmoniously in the mystery of my own Life.

The message from my unconscious has been very clear: Kath Wyatt's daughter has come home. Judith Wyatt / Nicholson has come home. Our new home in Mornington, as yet unnamed, is reminiscent of the Flinders "Binowee'; both have their own unique view out to sea. The Tumut "Binowee" also looked over water, down to the gurgling Goobragandra River, racing on its way to the sea. I have not been dumped, abandoned in Mornington. Things will continue to fall into place if only I can remember to be quietly, peacefully, trustingly and lovingly flowing in harmony with the Divine, myself and my world. Now that I finally understand this, will I be able to live this way? Only time will tell...

A Naked Soul

I have been quiet these last few weeks, doing very little of any moment, coming to terms in my own way, I suppose, with the tumultuous events of 11 September 2001. Will any of us ever forget that hauntingly beautiful spring day (here in southern Australia) and those incredible, unbelievable, horrifying images of death and destruction on our TV screens? Probably not.

The telephone woke me early that morning. I was deeply asleep dreaming that I was completely out of control and feeling so incredibly vulnerable with no possible way to protect myself. I stretched out an arm sleepily as the phone rang and heard Mark, whom I knew to be on the east coast of the United States of America, say, "Wake up Mum and turn on your TV." As I went to sit in front of the TV, Ian joined us on another phone; quietly together for a few minutes, we watched the reports of the horror unfolding. Yes, he was alright, Mark said, just deeply shocked. None of his friends had been physically harmed, although many, working in a building near the World Trade Centre, were traumatised by what they had witnessed.

On that day most of us were badly shaken. Suddenly we felt vulnerable; felt that never again would we have the same level of security. It was clear we would have to come to terms with this, each in our own way. It was also clear this would not be easy. These were feelings for all of us, nothing particular for me here. Why, then, nearly four weeks later do the images of those crumbling towers and billowing clouds of flames continue to haunt me, bringing tears, shivers and feelings of such vulnerability? For heavens sake I am one of the lucky ones, personally untouched by this tragedy, why am I so affected?

I pause for a minute trying to pull myself together. Is it possible the mirror of life is involved: that these images so powerful for all of us, are additionally reflecting to me something about my unconscious?[126] Certainly the feelings accompanying the imagery of crumbling structures and billowing flames are very intense, usually an indicator of unconscious material for me. And if I turn to my body, I find butterflies in my stomach as if I am anxious about an important event: a wedding, an exam or the diagnosis of a terminal illness perhaps. These are the ones I know from personal experience.

As I write my mind leaps and I see myself having a Rosen session with Gloria Hessellund late in 1997, about nine months after I left hospital for the last time following my treatment for leukaemia. Not long before, in a curious roundabout way, I had heard myself described in a Rosen context as "the administrator and sole Rosen practitioner in Australia". Suddenly on the table that morning come feelings of anger that those words, factual and objectively accurate as they were, in no way acknowledged my fundamental and continuing contribution to the Australian Rosen program.

Gloria, a sensitive and deeply intuitive Rosen practitioner asked a crucial question, "What do you feel the word "administrator" denies you, Judith, energy, commitment, passion?" *Passion* is the word; I feel it grab me as she says it. My passion for the unconscious and the body-mind continuum, my passion for Rosen Bodywork that facilitates that process, the passion that has fuelled these last thirteen years of my life since I began my training in 1988. That passion, I suddenly realise on the massage table, carried me through the loneliness and difficulties of being the sole Rosen practitioner in a huge country. Additionally it strengthened me as I battled the early administrative hassles of introducing a bodywork program into a society whose institutions were undoubtedly sceptical.

126 See *The Mirror of Life*, p. 153

In that same Rosen session with Gloria, my mind leapt and I saw myself back in the hospital in late 1996, hearing the leukaemia diagnosis and feeling so very naked. From the depths of her intuition, Gloria murmured the phrase "the naked soul" and suddenly together we were plumbing the depths of my unconscious. Again I saw myself in hospital now talking to one of the nurses of my passion for life. I saw clearly for the first time two Judiths: the sensible, rational woman I have known for decades; and now, emerging more recently as a result of all my Rosen work and my illnesses, a passionate one — a woman as yet not so well known. Again Gloria murmured, "The naked soul finds and honours passion, the core of Life, Life itself."

That session in 1997 changed gear, Gloria mentioned her puzzlement that she found my "responsibility muscles" so very much tighter than when she had given me a session earlier in the year just after I left hospital for the last time. "But, of course," I reply, "when I was in hospital I was so ill I lay surrounded by love, trustingly allowing the medical profession, my family and close friends to do whatever had to be done. I was not burdened by feelings of responsibility; I was simply living in love and trust. This was much easier in hospital than living my everyday life in the real world." And so that session came quietly to a close with one exquisite thought: the naked soul finds its passion, its life force and then lives its life in love and trust.

On reflection I think that passion has probably been an unacknowledged power in my life for many years. I now see passion in my early reaction to the unconscious which took me first to Rosen bodywork training and later to Tumut and the building of "Binowee" and the Australian Rosen program; passion too in my deep abiding love of books, my exploration of the world of ideas and now the writing of this book. Passion it seems has long been a part of my life, albeit until recently unacknowledged.

The message from that session with Gloria seems to be that a soul finds its individual passion and then lives its life in love and trust. Yet what does the word love mean in this context? Surely a naked, passionate soul can't be living its life in a love that carries connotations of dependence or need?[127]

Suddenly, I am reminded of a book I bought when travelling alone some years ago. Since it contained some nine hundred pages, I hoped it would fill many hours of solitary bus, train and plane travel.[128] It soon became apparent I had bought better than I knew, for in historical-novel form, it was a study of a medieval artist and the challenges to his artistic integrity. One passage describing the heroine contains a hauntingly beautiful phrase — "love was a field of action for her...not a need." To have love as a field of action, a place in which to operate with harmony, a place from which I move, but not a need. Ah that appealed to me. With love or its siblings — compassion and humanity — as fields of action I can offer the possibility of understanding, harmony and peace — all so very dear to my soul. Additionally, on a more personal level, I can freely explore the joys of my world without laying my vulnerable, sensitive soul open to rejection and pain. Freedom in love, freedom for love, freedom... love... What a lovely thought!

In June 2001 I visited California for the first time in ten years to attend a Rosen Retreat conducted by Marion Rosen herself and Elaine Mayland, one of her early collaborators and my teacher and supervisor during my training in Sweden. In a private Rosen session with Marion I asked her to look at my right buttock and hip saying they had been intermittently painful for years and I never seemed able to resolve the problem.[129] It must be wonderful to be eighty-seven, with a lifetime's wisdom, experience and skills to draw on. She worked for a few minutes and then remarked quietly, "Oh that buttock is pinched in with effort." *Effort*, the word sang throughout my body as I felt a muscle deep in my buttock release and images of a lifetime's efforts poured through my mind. We spoke together at the end of the session of the beauty of her work, its clarity, and its simplicity and its power.

From California I went first to London and then to Sweden where I found another of the wise women in my travels. After my five-year absence, Ingrid was once again welcoming me with open arms.

[127] See *Beloved, Ah beloved*, p. 141

[128] Edith Pargetter, *The Heaven Tree Trilogy*, Omnibus Edition, Warner Futura, London, 1994

[129] See *Death as a Friend*, p. 298. The pain in my hip had flared again on the move from Tumut, and on arrival in Mornington was worse than ever and obdurately refusing to shift. Medical tests showed that although there was some deterioration due to my age, of itself this should not be sufficient to cause the level of pain I was experiencing.

Apparently my right hip and buttock had more to say for they began to prickle as soon as she put her hands on my body. Gradually I felt the pressure building until suddenly a wave of muscular spasms travelled the full length of the right side of my body as muscle after muscle was released. Simultaneously I saw myself just born, naked, held aloft by my feet, as the doctor tapped my tiny bum and laughingly said, "You were a bit slow coming, weren't you? You couldn't have been trying hard enough." And then the ensuing lifetime always afraid of being late, and all that effort, all that effort...[130]

I know medical science would say that a tiny baby can't possibly have remembered and understood those words. I accept that. All I know is that sensible and normally to be trusted as I am, that session happened to me just exactly as I have described. I can only assume that my unconscious selected appropriate words to go with a childhood event (the very firm slap at birth) that was lying in the deepest level of my body and causing muscular tension. The results of that session combined with the one Marion gave me were stunning. The recurring pain in my hip and buttock that had bedevilled me increasingly for years had gone and so far shows so sign of return, (although I agree it may do so if I am tempted to put too much effort into anything).[131]

I also know that since I returned to Australia after these two Rosen sessions, it has been completely impossible for me to put any effort into anything. Just now I either do something because I want to, or I don't do it at all. I won't be able to live this way indefinitely; presumably balance will soon come drifting on the wind.

Why am I writing of this here, what has effort to do with the naked soul living in love? Recently I was talking to Jill of these two sessions and my inexplicable inability since my return to Australia to complete the few remaining pages of this book. "I don't understand, why I am so completely blocked," I said. She thought for a minute and then replied quietly "Perhaps you are feeling you have to finish it, whereas maybe you just need to feel you want to finish it." Ah, of course, *having* to finish it requires effort, whereas *wanting* to finish it does not.

[130] See *First Birthday*, p. 110

[131] In fact the pain in my right hip recurred about three months later in early 2002 and was then diagnosed as secondary breast cancer affecting the bones of my right hip and lower spine. See *A String of Pearls* p. 298

Effort, I began to understand, is not necessarily the physical exertion I put into an act, but a feeling I have when I am doing something I don't want to do. This explains why I can sometimes achieve seemingly arduous tasks without any "effort" and at others the smallest job seems impossible. This brings me back to love being a field of action and not a need. For if I want to do something, if I am acting out of love and not a need to be approved, to conform or to belong — any of the myriad shoulds, musts, oughts, and have tos — my desire to do it, my passion will be such that I won't feel any effort. What a lovely thought.

Trust was the other feeling that surfaced in that 1997 session with Gloria. The naked soul lives in love and trust. If you were to ask me whether I now manage to live in trust instead of attempting to control my every action, my first response would be to describe myself as the original doubting Thomas. "Trust", I cry, "don't know the word, not in my vocabulary." And yet as I write, I wonder, am I doing myself justice, or is my mind just replaying an old worn-out record it could be useful to discard? How would an outsider looking at my actions over the last ten years describe me — a trusting or non-trusting person? He or she would have to notice that I have blindly followed all those prompts from my meditation that bear a buzz of intensity, and would almost certainly describe me as trusting. So it could be that my lack of trust is only a devilishly demoralising feeling (like effort) that impedes the free flow of how I am trying to live my life.

I seem to have wandered far and wide today following — *trusting*! — that the promptings of my unconscious are leading me somewhere. What do images of crumbling towers and billowing flames have to do with my naked soul finding its passion and then living its life in love and trust? It is not difficult to correlate billowing flames and passion. But what is my unconscious trying to suggest with the metaphor of crumbling towers? Is it perhaps that my meditation, Rosen work and illnesses have weakened my previously fixed notion of my personality imposed by my then-unexplored conscious and unconscious minds (the concrete towers)? Until recently my ego with its fixed and well-known views has been protecting me, setting up defences and negative feelings, projecting much of what I didn't want to know of myself onto others, all the time hiding me not only from the world, but more importantly from myself. Now, though, with those structures greatly weakened, I am conscious of much more of myself (have raised my consciousness as the Yogis say), and am being offered the chance to live at least from time to time in contact with my naked soul. Is this why I feel so acutely vulnerable? I wonder...

For me the word *vulnerable* is negative, speaking of fear, pain and powerlessness in the face of strength. Yet, if I pause and look back I have often found relief from negative feelings by the substitution of positive ones: my love of mysteries instead of my fear of the unknown, my love of challenges instead of my feelings of being unable to cope. And the positive side of vulnerability must surely be sensitivity. My sensitivity has often brought pain, yet is something I have never been able to relinquish. Those feelings — call them vulnerability or sensitivity — like all else in the Universe, must be Divine, mustn't they? Is it what my ego experiences as vulnerability a God-given gift — an acute and subtle sensitivity, which is beginning to leave me full of wonder? It could well be...

So, if as a person stripped of many ego defences, I am being challenged to accept that vulnerability is also the gift of sensitivity, where will I find protection? As I write I have a glimmer of understanding. If from the depths of my soul, I can accept myself, move in harmony with myself, just exactly as I am — loving, generous, warm-hearted, intelligent and sensitive, yet prone to be anxious, insecure, feeling I'm wrong, seeking approval and vulnerable — if I can be at-one with myself without a whisper of movement "away from", that will be sufficient protection, won't it? For then there will be no chinks in my armour. This brings me to acceptance yet again. Self-acceptance this time. It is quite amazing how often variations on the theme of acceptance have surfaced in this book. Freedom it seems at base is comprised of acceptance in many guises.

Finally the World Trade imagery speaks not only of crumbling towers and passion, but also of danger, death and destruction. This seems to bring me to the two Judiths I spoke of earlier: the sensible, rational one and the passionate one. I am reminded of the one passage in Gibran's *Prophet* I love more than any other. Asked by the priestess to speak of reason and passion, Gibran replies: "Your reason and your passion are the rudder and sails of your seafaring soul."[132] Yes, of course, either on its own is capable of bringing about the destruction of the other, together with all I hold dear. I need both reason and passion, held in balance, harmony and integrity. Each will have its own appointed place in my life.

That phrase "seafaring soul" shows us another integral part of my naked soul. My passion, I would have to call it that, my passion for exploring, whether it is the physical world around me, the world of ideas, or most recently the metaphorical world of my unconscious and the related ideas of the body-mind continuum. There is no doubt, I love to explore, to live any other way is unthinkable. My seafaring, exploring soul — the Elephant's Child with his "satiable curtiosity."[133]

And so I am close to the end of my journey and as is the case in many myths and legends, I am nearing the place from which I started. Physically, after a lifetime's travels, I am back on the Mornington Peninsula, the land of my childhood. Yet like so many travellers I am returning infinitely richer. For I come bearing the treasures of my discovered soul: my deeply enriching and liberating self-knowledge, the many experiences on my spiritual journey, my joy in the small things of life — my family, reading, writing, teaching, swimming, walking in the woods, drinking coffee with friends, my joy in life itself in fact and what it brings me.

---

132 Khalil Gibran, *The Prophet*, p. 50

133 See *The Elephant's Child*, p. 9

The Angel of Pain[134]

Tears are running down my face; four times in the last nine years Ian and I have sat in doctors' surgeries and listened to cancer diagnoses — breast cancer, acute myeloid leukaemia, a major aggressive (but mercifully operable) cancer for Ian (and then in 2002 — I jump ahead — secondary breast cancer) for me. Four times we have heard the possible treatments, side effects, after effects and life expectancy. Four times we have returned home to make decisions and face the possibility of death.

There is a tremendous loss of innocence here, suddenly death is no longer an intellectual proposition, something that comes to everyone at the end of a long life; but real, sitting right there at the end of the bed, no longer sometime, but this year, next year... For me this has brought pain, anger, confusion, bewilderment: grief coming and going, ebbing and flowing like the tide; and tears, at first regular, expected, later spasmodic, unexpectedly triggered by some small thing. How do I, can I handle, manage, this pain?

There are differing reactions. As I answer the phone, I am crying, "I have the weeps this morning", I say to my caller. "Oh have you," she replies, and goes on with what she rang to say. She is one of the "not mes" of this world: "I don't want to know about your pain, nor do I want to

[134] In this tale I discuss the handling of the emotional pain involved in having cancer, a scene I know from personal experience. What I say can apply equally to all such pain. It is placed here so as not to interfere with the flow of the story of our last move and of the fourth cancer.

know about my own, not me." The not mes of this world won't listen to pain, turn rather to cigarettes, alcohol, parties, noise, golf, work, anything rather than face the painful reality. They have a following: people applaud them for returning quickly to work after surgery, ignoring the effects of radiation or chemotherapy and cancer itself. Is this courage, I wonder, or is it running away?

I lie in hospital crying quietly early one morning after the leukaemia diagnosis, a young Registrar visits, "Are you in pain, can I get you something?" he asks. "I have leukaemia, that's why I am crying," I reply. "Oh, of course, I'm sorry," he says. He is kind; he wants to comfort me by stopping my pain and offers me painkillers or tranquillisers — the only means available to him.

As Rosen students we were told repeatedly, "You mustn't comfort, you must not comfort." A really hard lesson to learn, if you don't deny someone's grief, then instinctively you want to lessen it by comforting. In a Rosen session, where a client comes to make contact with feelings, to comfort is to stop the flow of those feelings, to deny the purpose of the session. So no comforting. "You may cry as you give a session," I once heard Marion Rosen say, "only make sure your tears don't fall on your client!" Occasionally I do cry as I work; I hear some heart-rending stories, usually told for the first time.

Another problem with comforting is that the "poor you" sometimes implied in the comforter's voice and actions, may call forth "poor me". Oh poor me to whom all these dreadful things have happened; and "poor me", overindulged, is a weakening debilitating feeling. Who has the strength or courage to fight for survival while murmuring poor me! Poor me stands frozen, denied any chance of escape, irrevocably tied, bound, in hostage to the situation. Poor me...

I have a Rosen session with Gloria[135], and the cancer saga surfaces again. Tears flow, she works on quietly yet firmly, fingers probing gently, "What's this about Judith, and this?" I feel the compassion in her fingers, hear it in her voice, she won't run away from my grief; she won't stop the flow by comforting me; she will stand quietly listening to me, offering me

---

135 Gloria Hessellund, a gifted, sensitive and intuitive Rosen practitioner. As the Director of Teaching at the Berkeley Centre in California, she became the Director of Teaching in the Australian Rosen program on its sponsorship by the Berkeley Centre. After August 1996 Gloria and other Rosen teachers came regularly to Australia to conduct the intensive program and I was once again able to have regular Rosen sessions, although at long intervals.

the steadfast strength of her presence — compassion, the quiet courage to be with someone in pain.

Clearly in time of crisis I need comfort; similarly, at times denial seems the only option. However, if you assume, as I do, that cancer came into my life to bring me valuable experiences, to teach me something about my life I would not otherwise learn, how can I stay with it, not run away, and yet not fall into the easy trap of "poor me"? How can I manage to find compassion for myself wherever I might be? Enter the Angel of Pain...

In 1990, when Ian and I were travelling by car in northern Scotland seeking the erstwhile homes of the Nicholson clan, we visited Findhorn, a thriving educational centre on the shores of Moray Firth east of Inverness. Established by Peter and Eileen Caddy and Dorothy Maclean in 1962, it has grown from three adults and three children living in a caravan in a disused corner of a caravan park, to a community of 350 residents with over 5,000 visitors annually: all exploring meditation, healing in all its guises, craft, art, ecological balance and community living.

It was my mother who first gave me books about Findhorn in the late 1960s. A keen gardener, she liked to make a "matron's visit" around her garden each morning, checking on the health and well being of each of her plants. She was interested in Dorothy's work with plants. I, sparked initially by her interest, had over the years been more attracted to the many modalities of healing practised there. Now I had written ahead from Stockholm, telling of my training in bodywork and asking if it were possible to meet people working in related fields.

So it was that at Findhorn one Sunday morning, I was meditating with a small healers group: five or six of us were sitting in a circle, holding hands, gazing into the still flame of a candle. Words are too heavy, too limiting, to describe what followed; the experience was light, incredibly subtle, a fluttery touch, an instantaneous *knowing* that seemed to come from the whole of me. A Presence, if you like, brushed me with a light feathery stroke and simultaneously I *knew* the "Angel of Pain, love and compassion." Nothing negative, just wonderful positive feelings, loving, compassionate, tender, strong — everything one could possibly yearn for in the relief of pain; but, at the same time saying quietly, inexorably, pain is inevitable, every life contains pain at some stage, how else does growth occur.

The Angel of Pain — my treasure from Findhorn — I forget her at times and fall headlong into the traps of "poor me", occasionally "not me". Then, blocked in my life, treading the vicious treadmill of pain for whatever reason, I remember, Angel of Pain — love and compassion — and most importantly, love and compassion for myself. Herein lies the crux, love and compassion for myself, just exactly as I am, frightened of cancer treatments, frightened of the process of dying, grieving for the possible early loss of my life, furious with the Universe for putting me through this again. It's OK to be like that, but don't wallow in it — "poor me"; don't run away from it — "not me"; just stay there quietly with all the courage and strength you can muster, talk to the pain, explore it and see what this experience is bringing you, where it might take you.

For me to handle pain I found there were questions for which I wanted answers: in particular what is pain, where does it come from? Emotional pain often brings pain in the body, but not always. With my leukaemia, for instance, there was none of the physical pain one would associate with a burn, arthritis or an abscess; yet the emotional pain was acute, I could feel it tearing, ripping into me. I discovered on receiving the diagnosis that I loved life with a passion, I therefore did not want to die. So back and forth went my mind, was I going to die, when was I going to die, how was I going to die, what of my family, my unfinished book, the Rosen training program, my (to my mind) unfinished life? How could I live from day to day without knowing what the future held? Round and round went my mind, racing like a trapped mouse in a cage. When... what... how... when... what... how...?

Pain, say the Yogis, is a movement of the mind, a movement away, a twisting, tearing, a pulling away from "what is": a back and forth motion of the mind. Back into the past — if only I had, hadn't, I should have, should not have and so on. Forward into the future — where I was with leukaemia — "what if", endlessly. Nothing can now be done about most of the past, what was done, is done; no one knows what the future holds. Lessening, minimising the pain comes by trying to live in the present, this very moment of being, just being with whatever is. Over the years I have tried to seek a stillness, a state of being with the pain, no movement at all, let it come, let it go, just be at-one with it. My family would say that some days I manage this; on many others I come nowhere near it. But the Angel of Pain says this is a tough path, go gently, be kind to yourself...

Is acceptance a way to describe staying with pain? Every mainstream religion and most books on spiritual development talk of the need to accept those parts of ourselves and our lives that are immutable. Yet acceptance is a tricky concept for often it hides other feelings: we can apparently accept quietly and yet be "poor me", a victim of what life has done to us; or angrily becoming "not me" lose ourselves in some other pursuit; or with bitterness and resentment move to the "well I am jolly well stuck with this, so I'll bloody well have to make do," response. Each of these attitudes, although superficially acceptance, unconsciously contains other feelings — pain plus something else. In each of these states the mind has moved to victimisation, anger, resentment, in order to pick up, to "accept" the burden of the pain. None of this brings the peace of a truly quiet mind.

Ingrid used to say the Swedish word *forsoning* — in which there was no element of movement — more accurately reflected the state of mind we were seeking. Searching for an English equivalent, we came to the phrase at-one, to be at-one with the pain whatever it is, pain simpliciter: just to hang with it, be with it, move with it, disentangled from all other feelings. Then with what courage we can muster, we accept the challenge of a difficult situation and build it into the fabric of our lives.

How do you still the mind, be at-one with whatever it is that is bothering you? At the beginning of a crisis, when the mind is spinning almost out of control, this seems an impossible task. It quickly becomes evident, you don't decide *not* to think of cancer, death, divorce or abandonment. For consciously not to think of, is at the same time to think of; the word cancer is still in the mind. Some success can be had by diverting the mind whenever it starts its pain-laden cycle. I found the imagery of the surf beach at Merimbula helpful when I was in hospital with leukaemia, removing not only my mind, but as far as possible myself from the rigours of medical oncology at the Canberra Hospital, feeling the warm sand steadying me, the comfort of the sun's rays on my back, and allowing the rolling surf to have an almost hypnotic effect.

Nobody says this is easy, certainly not me: I manage on some days, not on others. One thing leads me on, the freedom involved: to try to accept life — to think and act in this way — brings freedom from pain, freedom from the fears and uncertainties of life. Freedom in fact to think of life as a gift — to think in terms of life as a miraculous gift — not a cross to be born. The Angel of Pain, love and compassion...

Dancing My Life

Death as a Friend, Trust and Other Pearls of Infinite Beauty

When I wrote the last tale, The Naked Soul, I thought my book, my tales of my travels in the world of my unconscious, my letters and reflections were finished, at least for the time being. Now some months later, I wonder how I could have been so naive, could have imagined that the story of those explorations could be complete without some personal understanding of what death might mean for me. And so, as I suppose I could have expected, my life organised itself once more so that death reappeared on the horizon.

Yes, my life has been turned upside down with yet another cancer diagnosis: my third brush with cancer in the last nine years. This time it was a secondary cancer arising from the breast cancer I had in 1993. Imagining I was free from that threat, I was stunned. Yet there was cancer lurking in the bones of my right hip and my lower spine and on the outer surfaces of both my lungs: an explanation of why I had felt so unwell during the summer of 2001-2002.

So with my wonderfully loving and supportive family and friends I went once again into cancer mode — radiation and drug therapy, overwhelming fatigue, tears, and the added burden of my body's intolerance of the recommended drugs. I have been very ill.

It is not of pain and suffering that I wish to write this morning, I have already done that,[136] but of trust, the most wondrously exquisitely beautiful feeling to come my way. Hold me in your heart while I try to tell you my continuing story of trust. It comes not so much as a logical chronological tale but rather as a series of vignettes, little cameos of experience, *my pearls...*

The horrors of this cancer hit me one really bad day in May 2002. Suffering the combined after-effects of radiation for bone cancer and my body's intolerance of the drugs, I was as ill as I have ever been. In effect I told Ian I just wanted to lie down and die. "It's too much", I said, "I just can't handle my life any longer, I'm off."" People talk of "battling" with cancer; but I was way beyond that. I have written at length of "accepting" cancer, but I was way beyond that also, for acceptance requires my agreement — a movement from me however slight. That morning I felt completely incapable of doing any single thing. I was surrendering completely to my life, my death, or whatever else the Universe had to offer — an utter abject surrender[137]. To my great surprise surrender eased the trauma of that morning and brought feelings of some peace. So here is my first and most unlikely pearl — *surrender.*

One of the more difficult aspects of any secondary cancer is that it can only be managed or controlled by treatment. Of itself it is ineradicable. Initially I found this hard. I had to come to terms with a conscious ever-present awareness that this cancer, although not of itself life threatening, could strike again at any time, all this might mean for me in terms of ill health, a total disruption of my life as I like to live it, and possible death.

Now try as I may to disassociate cancer from death, I find it almost impossible. I know this particular cancer is not supposed to be life threatening and I know that I have already recovered from two earlier cancers. A new acquaintance jokingly remarked recently: "You seem to have more lives than a cat!" And yet, and yet, despite all the logic and all my commonsense, in my mind and the minds of most twenty-first century people, there is little doubt that cancer and death are virtually synonymous. A cancer diagnosis is for some people a death sentence and,

---

[136] See *The Angel of Pain*, p. 292

[137] I realised later that when I had leukaemia I was not so much accepting, as bargaining with Death, saying, "You let me lead the life I like to lead for however short a time, and I will agree to die when You want me to." This time I had no strength for negotiation.

for those who do not die, their first personal experience of their mortality.

I spoke of death one day to a young acupuncturist friend. "How can I come to terms with living so close to death?" I wondered. His reply turned my question on its head. "Oh," he said quietly, "in a way I envy you, I have no personal knowledge of death and the thought of it terrifies me. I would love to be able to live close to death, *to know death as a friend*." Death as a friend, the phrase haunted me for days, how would it be to have death as a friend. How indeed? Another pearl, perhaps…?

Then wandering the house one sleepless night, an insight floated up from the depths of my unconscious and my mind leapt sidewards. Death, I suddenly saw, was not the end of life, but an integral part of it. Paradoxically, without death there could be no life; similarly without life there could be no death. The existence of each was inextricably dependent on the existence of the other. In the world of the conscious mind, a world of separation, definition and duality, in which we define death as the end of physical life as we know it, such an insight appears nonsensical. Yet that insight came from my unconscious and brought with it such feelings of peace and clarity — death as an inseparable part of life, death as a part of the Life I love so much. *Death as a friend*…another pearl, one of indescribable beauty this time.

A few days later I was having a massage and the topic of death came up again. "What does the word death mean to you?" the masseuse asked. With barely a moment's pause and without any reflection, the answer came straight from my unconscious, "My physical body may disintegrate and stop functioning," I replied, "but my soul, or whatever word you like to use, some part of me, continues living through eternity. This I know from the very depths of my being." *Eternal life*, another pearl…

Since death and cancer seem to be so closely entwined for me, if I am to think of death as a friend, it is clear I will need to have more positive thoughts about cancer. I need to see it not in terms of the possible end of my life. I need to look beyond pain — be it physical or emotional — effort and disruption and frustration. A session at the Gawler Cancer Foundation helped me but it is the frustration I now find so hard, I think.

In a quite diabolical way cancer interrupts how I want to live my life. Three times I have planned my life with all the things I know I really wanted to do. Bang, I have a cancer diagnosis, and it all has to be put aside for however long it takes me to recover. Although I do keep recovering, I know what cancer treatments do to my sensitive body, and the effort I have to make to regain my strength and take my place in the non-cancer world again.

It appears then, that to make death (and its mate-by-association, cancer) my friends, I need to start by trying to use a less fearsome word than cancer in my thoughts. I was driving along a beautifully treed road one day floating with these ideas, when the word *teacher* drifted up: what if I were to regard cancer, not so much as possible death or, at the least, an unwelcome interruption in my life, but as a teacher? Soothed and steadied by the surrounding beauty, I looked back down the last nine years of my life. Yes, there had been much cancer, but every where I looked I saw the insights and the understanding my cancer experiences had brought. It was no exaggeration to call cancer a teacher, my teacher; it was no more than the truth. As I shifted in my thoughts from cancer-equals-death mode to cancer-equals-teacher mode, I felt my tension and fears easing — a recognition of the *power of the mind*, another pearl of inestimable value…

Over the years, sceptics have hinted that my recurrent cancers don't support my thesis that exploration of my unconscious has helped in my recovery. They wonder, if perhaps the cancers recur because I did not deal previously with all "my issues". That could be, none of us can know. As I see it, I have dealt with whatever feelings arose. Some came in one cancer experience and some in the next. See what happens, though, if I regard cancer as a teacher. Then it is as if a teacher is saying, "This — death — is a complex subject. You won't be able to handle it all at once. So I will give it to you slowly piece by piece, allowing you time for reflection and integration."

One beautiful late summer's morning in February 2003, it was a little misty, cool and quietly sunny. From nowhere, over the past few weeks have come beautiful feelings of trust. I have written before of trust in *Shackles*.

Such a simple little word I wrote, such a slippery, elusive customer. "Blessed are they that trust," I said, "they will surely inherit the earth, warm, loving, joyous, carefree, spontaneous people. Would that we all might be..."[138] *Trust*, I am discovering brings feelings I had never previously known — deep abiding joy and a beauteous quiet all-pervading feeling of safety. Pearls of infinite beauty...

Intellectually I can speculate that feelings of trust have now floated to the surface of my life because I no longer fear death.[139] I said earlier in this book that I did not think I feared death. I now realise that there was an ever-present undercurrent of anxiety of which I was not even aware until it was no longer present. Does this make sense? Only by its absence do I become aware of its previous presence. I can speculate even further and say that this anxiety was triggered by my love of life and my fear that it was coming to a close earlier rather than later.

These, however, are but intellectual games. What I really want to do this morning is to wonder at the glory of trust. For I discover that it permeates everywhere, touches and transforms every facet of the jewel that is my life. For I have discovered that for me trust is the most basic of all feelings. If I trust, I will have the strength and the courage to handle difficult situations. If I trust, I will have compassion, patience, serenity, balance. If I trust I can offer love, one of the most precious gifts in my life, without feeling vulnerable and fearing rejection.

Moreover trust offers me the chance to handle my life without effort, to live without strain, without the need to control or to limit, an opportunity to flow with the stream of my life, to dance to the music that is my life — whatever metaphor you wish to use. Last year, far from well, I went to see one of the world's great ballerinas dance the title role in *Giselle* — one of the Western world's greatest classical ballets. I sat entranced, never have I seen such effortless, floating dancing as in her portrayal of a ghostly wraith. Would that I could live my life that way...

Trust also takes me to the inexplicable mysteries of my life: I trust myself even if I do not fully understand how I am as I am. It enables me to accept that at one and the same time I am both frightened of the

---

[138] See "*Shackles*" at p. 42

[139] See *Land of Confusion*, p. 258

unknown and yet love mysteries, that I can still be rattled by the I-can't-cope syndrome and yet love challenges, that freedom is all in all to me and yet paradoxically involves acceptance, that I am responsible for my own life and yet part of the Divine over which I can have no control.

I no longer have my beautiful Goobragandra River as a source of inspiration, but I do have the glories of Port Phillip Bay, the ever-changing beauty of light on water. The beauty of the harmony, the balance, the totally spontaneous flow of life, each part moving freely, apparently without direction, yet precisely in its own place — the dance of life. We are each part of this dance, dancing the stories of our lives: sad, happy, peaceful or angry, dancing to the music of Life. The Dancer Within...

And so my story is finished.

Epilogue

Though said not to be life threatening, Judith's recurrence of breast cancer after nine years spread and spread. It could not be managed by radiotherapy or chemotherapy. She could not tolerate the drugs prescribed, as most others do, perhaps because her immune system had been weakened by leukaemia.

Judith died quietly and peacefully in hospital in July 2004, surrounded by her loving family, who, in accordance with her wishes, have published this, her book.

Bibliography

Bible, King James version, Cambridge University Press, Cambridge,

de Mello, Anthony, SJ, *The Song of the Bird*, Image, Doubleday, New York, 1984

Clift, Wallace B., *Jung and Christianity, The Challenge of Reconciliation*, Collins Dove, Victoria, Australia, 1983

Dessaix, Robert, *Night Letters*, Macmillan, Sydney, 1996

Fox, Mathew, *The Coming of the Cosmic Christ*, Harper & Row, San Francisco, 1988

Franklin, Joy and Mary-Margaret Moore (eds) *Bartholomew, Reflections of an Elder Brother*, High Mesa Press, New Mexico, 1990

Gibran, Kahlil, *The Prophet*, William Heinemann, London, 1980

Hay, Louise L., *Heal Your Body*, Specialist Publications, Sydney, 1986

Hammarskjold, Dag, *Markings*, Faber and Faber, London, 1988

Heisenberg, Elisabeth, *Inner exile: Recollections of a Life with Werner Heisenberg*, translated by S. Cappellari and C. Morris, Birkhauser, Boston, 1984

Jung, C. G., *Dreams*, ARK edition, London, 1991

Jung, C. G., *Memories, Dreams and Reflections*, Flamingo, London, 1985

Jung C. G. & Wilhelm Reich, *The Body As Shadow*, John P. Conger, North Atlantic Books, California, 1988

Jung, C. G., *Four Archetypes: Mother, Rebirth, Spirit, Trickster*, ARK Edition, London, 1986

Jung, C. G., *Analytical Psychology Its Theory and Practice*, ARK edition, London1986

Jung, C. G. and Teresa of Avila, *Spiritual Pilgrims,* Book by John Welch, Paulist Press, New York, 1982

Jung, C. G., *Man and his Symbols*, Picador, London, 1978

Jung, C. G., *Psychology & Religion*, Yale University Press, 1938

Kipling, Rudyard, *Just So Stories*, Harper Collins, New York, 1996

Loades, Ann, *Dorothy L. Sayers: Spiritual Writings*, SPKC, Great Britain, 1993

Macquarie Dictionary, Macquarie Library Pty Ltd, McMahons Point, Australia, 1982

Mayland, Elaine L., *Rosen Method: An Approach to Wholeness and Well-being through the Body*, Private Publication, 8th Ed. 1996

McGuire, William and R. F. C Hull (eds), *C. G. Jung Speaking: Interviews and Encounters* Picador, London, 1980

Modjeska, Drusilla, *Poppy*, McPhee Gribble, Penguin Books Australia Ltd., 1990

Nicholson, Judith A, 'Changing Course: A Leap from Law to Bodywork', *Temenos: An Australian Jungian and Cultural Review*, Issue 2, Spring 1995, p. 44

Nicholson, Judith A., "Rosen Method Bodywork: A Newcomer to Australia", *The Natural Therapist*, Volume 13, No.1, 1998, p. 4

Pargetter, Edith, *The Heaven Tree Trilogy*, Omnibus Edition, Warner Futura, London, 1994

Rilke, Rainer Maria, *Letters to a Young Poet*, Joan M. Burnham (Trans.), New World Library, Novato CA., 1992

Rosen, Marion & Sue Brenner, *Rosen Method Bodywork: Accessing the Unconscious through Touch*, North Atlantic Books, Berkeley, California, 2003

Sandford, John A., *Healing and Wholeness*, Paulist Press, New York, 1977

Teerguarden, Iona Marsaa, *Acupressure Way of Health: Jin Shin Do*, Japanese Publications, Inc., 1978

Whitmont, Edward C., *The Symbolic Quest*, Princeton University Press, Princeton, 1978